Alkaline Ketogenic Lifestyle for Massive Weight Loss

Eat Your Way to Unstoppable Energy and a Sexy, Healthy Body without Feeling Bored or Deprived!

By Elena Garcia
Copyright Elena Garcia © 2020

Sign up for new books, fresh tips, super healthy recipes, and our latest wellness releases:

www.YourWellnessBooks.com

All rights reserved. No part of this publication may be reproduced, stored in a retrieval system, or transmitted, in any form or by any means, electronic, mechanical, photocopying, recording or otherwise, without the prior written permission of the author and the publishers.

The scanning, uploading, and distribution of this book via the Internet or via any other means without the permission of the author are illegal and punishable by law. Please purchase only authorized electronic editions, and do not participate in or encourage electronic piracy of copyrighted materials.

Disclaimer

A physician has not written the information in this book. It is advisable that you visit a qualified dietician so that you can obtain a highly personalized treatment for your case, especially if you want to lose weight effectively. This book is for informational and educational purposes only and is not intended for medical purposes. Please consult your physician before making any drastic changes to your diet.

All information in this book has been carefully researched and checked for factual accuracy. However, the author and publishers make no warranty, expressed or implied, that the information contained herein is appropriate for every individual, situation or purpose, and assume no responsibility for errors or omission. The reader assumes the risk, and full responsibility for all actions and the author will not be held liable for any loss or damage, whether consequential, incidental, and special or otherwise, that may result from the information presented in this publication.

The book is not intended to provide medical advice or to take the place of medical advice and treatment from your personal physician. Readers are advised to consult their own doctors or other qualified health professionals regarding the treatment of medical conditions. The author shall not be held liable or responsible for any misunderstanding or misuse of the information contained in this book. The information is not intended to diagnose, treat, or cure any disease. It's merely an inspiration to live a healthy lifestyle. If you suffer from any medical condition, are pregnant, lactating, or on medication, be sure to talk to your doctor before making any drastic changes in your diet and lifestyle.

Table of Contents

Alkaline Ketogenic Combo for Massive Weight Loss 7
    Optimizing Your Weight Loss and Health Success the Right Way 20
    How Not to (Keto) Diet 23
The 3 Missing Factors to Permanent and Healthy Weight Loss 27
    Pillar #1 Use Good Fats to Lose Weight (aka the Keto Secret Paradox) 27
Coconut Oil Tips & Recipes to Eliminate Sugar Cravings 32
    Coconut Oil Cortado Style Coffee Recipe 32
    Creamy Cinnamon Latte Recipe 33
    Green Tea Weight Loss Drink 34
    Creamy Coconut Ice Cream Recipe 35
More Simple Recipes to Feed Your Body with Some Good Fats! 36
    Spicy Avocado Smoothie 36
    Anti-Stress Infusion 37
    Cashew Nut Crew Snacks 37
    Egg Butter Avocado Breakfast or Brunch 38
    The 5 Ingredient 5 Minute Salad 39
    Easy Mediterranean Tuna Salad 40
    Weight Loss Pillar #2 Alkaline Autopilot for Smooth Weight Loss and Effortless Keto Lifestyle 49
    The Most Common Keto Mistakes 50
    The Alkaline Lesson #1 – You Need Alkaline Minerals 52
Understanding the Alkaline Diet to Lose Weight and Keep It Off 59
    Natural and Sustainable Weight Loss 59
    Energy, Improved Mood + Increased Motivation on the Alkaline Diet . 59
    Increased Health, Balance, and Vitality 60
    Mental Focus on the Alkaline Diet 61
    Detox 61

Going Alkaline in an Easy Way 62

It's NOT about RAISING or changing your pH 62

Is Alkaline Diet Hard to Follow? 67

What are alkaline foods? Is it about their pH? 67

Weight Loss Pillar #3 Right Food Lists, Right Mindset & Easy Recipes You Will Love! 71

Your alkaline-keto-friendly food lists 72

Alkaline Keto Meal Plans and Recipe Templates 86

Alkaline Keto Salad Recipe Template 91

Alkaline Keto Smoothie Template 92

Alkaline Keto Juice and Drink Template (no juicer needed) 92

Warm Alkaline Keto Recipe Template 93

Alkaline Keto Recipes Made Super Easy! 94

Easy Low Carb Pizza Adventure 94

Servings: 2 94

Irresistible Veggie Pizza 96

Easy Chili Tea 97

Cumin and Caraway Tea 98

Easy Flavored Spinach Juice 99

Red Bell Pepper Antioxidant Juice 100

Easy Chilly Beetroot Soup 101

Spicy Creamy Coconut Dream 102

Anti-Inflammatory Ginger Soup 103

Light Alkaline Keto Juice 104

Apple Cider Antioxidant Juice for Optimal Energy 105

Herbal Weight Loss Juice 107

Amazing Keto Chocolate Shake 108

Ridiculously Easy Sweet Alkaline Keto Balls 109

Creamy Sweet Alkaline Keto Porridge ... 110
Smoked Salmon Green Salad ... 111
Easy Mediterranean Baby Spinach Salad ... 112
Cucumber Creamy Green Smoothie ... 113
Boost Your Brain Smoothie ... 114
Cheesy Pumpkin Surprise ... 115
Alkaline Green Keto Energy Salad ... 116
Healing Herbs Avocado Salad ... 117
Ketoricious Energy Smoothie ... 118
Herbal Wellness Smoothie ... 119
The Supermodel Glow Smoothie ... 120
Easy Spicy Papaya Salad ... 121
More Alkaline Keto Books ... 122

Alkaline Ketogenic Combo for Massive Weight Loss

Thank you so much for taking an interest in this book. It really means a lot to me!

I am very excited to be sharing this weight loss guide with you. In fact, if you follow through and stay committed to it, this could be the last weight loss book you will ever read, seriously!

My intention behind writing this book is simple. I want to create something that was easy-to-follow and, at the same time, doable and fun for an average busy person.

I also wanted to create something that can help you achieve your weight loss goals as soon as possible, in a way that is healthy and sustainable.

It is my sincere desire that this book helps you transform your lifestyle and completely change the way you think about your diet and your body.

There will be no fluff and no unnecessary fillers. This book is designed to be read in one sitting (or 2) shall you choose to do so. Also, this is not your typical coffee-table book. What matters to me are your results. I don't write to be famous. I write to share what has worked for me to help you achieve your weight loss goals in a way that is healthy and effective (and as fast as possible).

So, my question to you is – *how badly do you want it? Are you ready to commit to a lifestyle change, right here and right now?*

Are you ready to give yourself the freedom to feel confident, healthy, and empowered?
Are you ready to let go of the old and embrace the new? Do you value your weight loss results? Are you sick and tired of a vicious cycle of diets that don't work?

Do you sometimes feel like you are losing your motivation because, nothing in the past has seemed to work?

Perhaps you are feeling skeptical thinking: *Will this help? Is it worth it? What if it doesn't work?*

Whatever is going on in your head right now, I get it, because I have been there myself! And I know one thing for sure – most of us, I mean, people who read books like this one, do it because they want results and transformation. I guess that you don't just want to sit and read diet and weight loss books or some nutritional guides for fun! Unless you are passionate about reading, recipes, or nutrition. But, for most of us, we get diet books because we want to get results. We want to see the results and feel good about ourselves. We also want others to see how much weight we have lost. For good. Once and for all!

I remember my frustration...reading a diet book after a diet book. I was joining expensive weight loss programs. And I was feeling very frustrated and demotivated when they didn't work.

I would then read books on motivation and discipline. So that I could "stick to a diet" and be successful. And while I did learn a lot from those self-help books, I still had nothing to show for, and I felt stupid.

I felt like a loser, like a follower and a self-help and diet junkie with no results. I had all those bits and pieces and had no idea how to turn them into a system that worked.

It took me 10 years of research and experimentation (and thousands of dollars, if not a 5 figure number spent on pills, books, programs, and other tools that did not work) to come up with a simple, 3-step-weight-loss-system that anyone could benefit from! Right now, as a weight loss and wellness writer, I am on the other side – it is my job to help you, the reader!

I am feeling very grateful for my weight loss journey, the good and the bad, because I can now relate to you, my friend. I know what it's like to spend money and time on things that don't work, are not sustainable, require you to give up your social life forever, spend 3 hours a day in the gym, do some unrealistic cleanses, take expensive supplements, and who knows what.

But now I am grateful for everything I have tried, even things that did not work.

My grandma used to say – *You don't fail. You succeed, or you learn.* And boy, was she right! The things that did not work made me stronger. Also, now I know what to avoid, and I am confident I can drastically shorten your weight loss journey and lead you straight to the results you want.

Years ago, when I was trying to lose weight unsuccessfully (or I could not keep it off, which was also very frustrating!), I made a promise to myself.

The promise was simple: Elena, as soon as you find the way to lose weight and keep it off, you will write about it and share it with other people to make sure they avoid your early mistakes (and save money and time!). You will do it with no hype and no false promises. Instead, you will give your people a proven blueprint they can use to get the results they are after, step-by-step, as fast as possible.

There is nothing wrong with fast weight loss, as long as the methods that lead to it are healthy and balanced! While certain levels of patience are required, it doesn't have to take you years to start losing weight. You can start feeling lighter in just a few days, and then, keep getting predictable results week after week (until your perfect body weight is achieved).

Imagine how good it will feel to get the results you want and start feeling great in your body! Now, in order to make your weight loss journey easy, enjoyable, and fun (and as effective as possible), it's crucial you focus on what really matters and release all the negative emotions (and disappointment) about losing weight.

Preparation is key to success, so give yourself the gift of learning to make sure your journey is easy and enjoyable (once again, losing weight doesn't have to be hard, if you have the right tools, system and the mindset – precisely what this book teaches!).

So, turn off your phone and eliminate distractions. Promise yourself to read this book as soon as you can, but don't just skip through it, hoping to find some "missing secrets" to weight loss. Release all your skepticism. Allow yourself to truly understand the 3 missing pillars to weight loss that this book covers.

Also, to give you some peace of mind (stress and weight loss are not the best friends).

This book is not a strict diet plan that you "have to follow". So you don't need to worry about picking up a start date and feeling worried or stressed that maybe some family occasions come up and you will "get off track". There is no more worrying that: "OMG, I am starting tomorrow, and I need to get all the ingredients to do my diet, but I also need to make sure I cook for my children or husband." The recipes you will find at the end of this book are husband and boyfriend (and also kids) approved. So, you can relax! Yes, there will be food lists and the flexible meal plans at the end of the book. But all of them will revolve around the 3 simple weight loss pillars (aka the missing factors to sustainable weight loss, almost on an autopilot).

All the diet and lifestyle changes can be taken gradually. And, each pillar will tell you exactly what to eat more of and what to eat less of.

Also, for the purpose of this book and your results, you don't have to think about going into ketosis or measuring your pH. Nothing wrong about that, but, it's not necessary for you to do to help you get the weight loss results that you want.

Pretty good stuff, isn't it?

The approach you are just about to discover is flexible so that you can create the perfect balance without feeling deprived or "over-dieting," but also without overindulging in foods you know are not good for you (so that you don't feel like a failure).

Instead, you will be giving your body the best foods (as well as drinks and mindsets) to help it start losing weight for you and even boosting your mood in the process!

Heck, you are not even required to count your calories or macros. Don't get me wrong; it is a smart thing to do, especially if you have some specific fitness goals in mind or are an athlete.

But, it can be quite a hustle for an average busy person, who works full-time and has family obligations.

So, once again, this book does not require any calorie counting or strict dieting.

Its flexible approach is deeply rooted in common-sense. For example, if you overthink the whole thing, and give yourself way too many guidelines to stick to (trying to be all perfect all at once), chances are you will get off track (and back to "guilt-trips" or feeling like "other people can do it but I can't!").

On the other side of the spectrum, "flexible" doesn't mean overindulging in some ridiculous cheat days filled with fast food. It's all about balance! This is exactly what the clean food, alkaline-keto approach is all about.

The 3 pillars are all interconnected. However, they do not need to be followed in any specific order. From my experience, the easiest way to go through them is by sticking to the order outlined in this book.

Also, the weight loss pillars we will be using are backed up by science. The reason why I mention this is that alkaline, as well as keto diets, often get a bad rep. The alkaline diet for being a quackery pseudo-science diet and keto for being a controversial diet that goes totally against the standard food pyramid.

So, it's normal that you might be feeling skeptical. But you see- these diets only get a bad rep because of greedy individuals who misuse those diets to make unrealistic (and very often medical) claims to get money from vulnerable people.

However, as soon as we will dive into the real essence of the alkaline diet (which is NOT about changing your pH) and keto diet (which has been used in medical settings for dozens of years and is the most effective diet to help you get rid of sugar and carb cravings), you will quickly understand that both diets take a very simple, common-sense approach to wellness and health.

(I will also be including some authoritative books and research on both diets, in case you're one of those nerds, like myself, who enjoys reading this stuff).

But, if all you want is to lose weight relatively fast – don't worry about all those "diet labels." This book will show you the practical how so that you know what to do to lose weight.

My simple, 3 pillar system is based on a few simple tweaks you can easily apply to your diet, lifestyle, and even mindset. No metaphysics and no "woo-woo". I will give you a very practical and science-backed mindset tips to help you stay on track and never worry about motivation again!

Alkaline Keto Lifestyle for Massive Weight Loss

By applying the 3 weight loss pillars outlined in this book, you will be finally able to:
-melt away up to 30 pounds of fat (while still enjoying nice, creamy, and fatty meals!)
-balance your blood sugar (prevention is the best cure!)
-potentially decrease the risk of many diseases and boost your immune system
-ease joint pain and feel more energized

Without over-dieting and over-exercising.

I have already covered our mindset around flexibility. Now, it's time to address the exercise.

Readers always ask me: *Do I really have to exercise? I hate it and I don't have the time to go to the gym.*

Well, here's the truth- the answer is both *yes* and *no*.
Or perhaps, I should have said: I have bad news and good news. Which news shall I share first?

OK, let's do the bad news first...
Many diet books, health coaches, and nutritionists will use the "Oh, you don't have to exercise, just do my diet, and you will lose weight without having to exercise" as a "hook" to get you to their programs. It's a marketing tactic.

Wow, I can lose weight without having to exercise!
Finally, someone gets me. Let me buy this new program!

OK, so now that I have covered the bad news...yes, you will have to do some physical exercise to speed up your weight loss success, tone up your body, and get rid of loose skin and cellulite (an unwanted weight loss surprise!).

Once again, the "No exercise is required team" will get you covered in their weight loss programs. They will upsell you a myriad of pills, ointments, and capsules to fight loose skin and cellulite.

What they say to "help you" is based more on their marketing and upsell schedule rather than on your actual weight loss success backed up by a good mood, and a healthy, fit and sexy body. **Here's the GOOD NEWS, though...**

While exercise is necessary to speed up your weight loss journey, make you feel confident and more energized (and as healthy as possible), **you don't need to OVEREXERCISE!**

This is exactly what I covered in one of my earlier promises...**You don't need to over-exercise, and it doesn't have to be all or nothing.**

Also, you don't have to go to the gym, and it's not necessary to workout for hours every day (unless you really enjoy your physical activity). Exercise can be free, almost effortless, and fun.

You need to move your body to get rid of toxins and stimulate your lymphatic system (as well as to avoid the above-mentioned loose skin and possibly cellulite).

Many of you dislike the idea of working out, because you feel disconnected from your body, or you think people will judge you. I have been there. I remember signing up for the gym, feeling so motivated. And the first day, someone called me a fatty. I felt so miserable and nearly lost all my hope. I thought, wait, is the gym only for slim and fit people? Everyone needs to start somewhere! So, I kept going. I actually turned all my negative feelings into motivation.

Someone called me a fattie, wait I will show them! But here's the thing. My goal was simple: 30 minutes of cardio, 3-5 times a week. It was easy to stick to. I noticed my mood was better, I slept better, my diet was easier, I binged on unhealthy foods much less, and I just felt good about exercising.

Eventually, I joined a group walking classes in my local gym, and then I also tried a few bodyweight classes. And I thought to myself, wait, I can do this by myself, at home! I don't need to pay for the gym now!

And so, I looked up bodyweight exercises online and began working out at home. Driving to the gym and preparing my gym bag, and everything turned out to be a bit time-consuming. So, the ability to work out at home gave me more freedom and flexibility.

The best part? I used to pay for the gym, drive there, and do cardio exercises or spinning. However, after I switched to body weight exercises (only 5-15 minutes a day, 4-5 times a week), I noticed much better results. And I didn't have to pay to work out.

Now, whatever works for you- do it. Some people need to pay for the gym to stay more motivated, or perhaps they just get pumped seeing other people working out.

But for me, bodyweight exercises at home were a big life changer! They are the quickest way to tone up your body, and also speed up the fat burn. I just found this method way more effective than long cardio sessions.

Now, it's time for a bit of tough love!
If you're still thinking you don't have the time to work out.
Let me ask you - how much time do you spend scrolling on your phone? What if you use your phone to watch bodyweight sessions and follow through them?

Trust me! You will lose weight faster, and you will feel amazing. After all, you want results, right? You want the transformation! Just stay consistent. Fifteen minutes a day, from home, is not an overwhelming goal!

As I said- what we want to avoid is over-exercising. At the early stage of my journey, I used to think I could eat fast food and a ton of crappy carbs and sugars just by over-exercising. It worked at first (the calories in and calories out theory, plus, I was young and pretty healthy).

But, unfortunately, eventually, it made me very sick. Unhealthy diet, fitness supplements, fat burn pills, energy drinks that would overstimulate my body did not lead to healthy and sustainable weight loss. Instead, I was always very sick and eventually ended up with adrenal exhaustion.

Well, at least I learned my lesson! Balance is the key to everything, and no amount of exercise can help balance out the side effects of a poor, Western, processed, and fast-food diet!

So, to sum up- to make the Alkaline Ketogenic Lifestyle more effective, add some moderate exercise you enjoy. It can be bodyweight, yoga, walking (I love walking in nature while listening to some inspiring audiobooks!), dancing, pilates, swimming, hiking....whatever you prefer.

It doesn't have to be all or nothing. Commit to something you enjoy and allow yourself to do it. Don't listen to gurus who tell you you don't need to exercise, but, at the same time, don't torture yourself with over-exercising. Pick up some activity to move your body and commit to it!

Oh...and when it comes to getting weight loss and wellness advice. Always ask yourself if a given guru tells you what you want to hear (so that it's easier for them to sell you stuff, that, most likely, you don't need), or what you actually need to hear to help you reach your goals (most often, it's harder to market).

Well, I only hope you don't hate me for telling you that we need some exercise to make it as effective as possible. As fast as possible, while still keeping it as healthy as possible.

Make sense?

Also, something is better than nothing. For example, 5 minutes of exercise is better than no exercise at all. So, whenever you don't have the time to exercise, or you don't feel like it, set a simple goal you can follow. Even 1 minute can be a massive shift for your mind (suddenly it will think: *Oh wow, we always follow through our goals!*). In other words, you will feel more confident, knowing that you can trust yourself and love yourself, without having to be 100% perfect.

So, why don't you get up and exercise for a minute? Just to get back to it and remind yourself how good it feels to move your body.

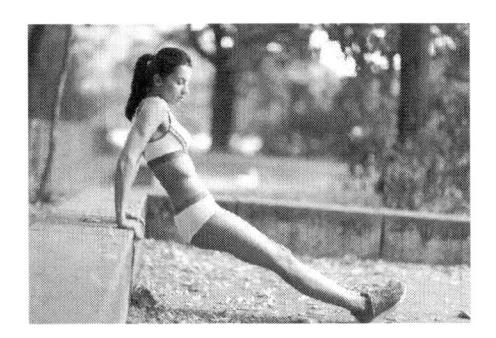

Optimizing Your Weight Loss and Health Success the Right Way

If you are already eating healthy and clean- you will learn how to take it to the next level, just by making a few simple tweaks to your diet and lifestyle.

And if you are just getting started on healthy living and natural, sustainable weight loss, this program will help you save months, if not years, of your life, so that you can focus on what works instead. So, if you are still on a SAD, Western diet, and have no clue where to start, don't worry, I have been there too, and we are in this together!

Now, I know that the intro is a bit long here, but if you want to be successful with this program, you need to understand the right mindset behind it. No, I am not a self-help guru or expert, and I am not here to tell you how to live your life. Instead, I want you to focus on what matters to you- fast and healthy weight loss results that last!

Before writing this book, I asked myself- what do all my successful readers and friends, I mean people who lost weight using this program, have in common?

-Do they always wake up full of motivation?
-Do they have hours of free time a day for endless shopping and complicated cooking?
-Are they the most disciplined and will-powered humans ever?
-Are they 100% perfect with their diet all the time? Are they ultra keto, carefully scrutinizing all the macros, or hardcore alkaline,

*trying to survive on salads alone? (*if you are new to this, no worries, we will be diving into keto and alkaline explanations soon!*)*.

And it dawned on me. All my successful readers and friends just took action and trusted the process. They took massive imperfect action and kept going. And none of them was 100% perfect with their diets. They committed and did the best they could while gradually transitioning to a healthy alkaline ketogenic lifestyle designed to lose weight.

The "keyword" here is: GRADUALLY!
I remember talking to one of my newsletter subscribers who kept postponing her lifestyle change. First, it was a holiday. Then, it was a new job. Then, some family occasions. And so, she would never start.

And I don't blame her. The old way of dieting and losing weight is based around being 100% perfect, getting some restrictive diet plan, and sticking to it, with no room for flexibility.

The good news? With this book, you can start making sustainable changes to your diet, even if you're going on a holiday tomorrow or your cousin is getting married next weekend.

The best time to start is always now, and it doesn't have to be all or nothing. Feels so good, doesn't it?

Most of my successful readers and friends were able to lose 20, 30, or even 100 pounds by merely switching most of their foods, meals, and drinks to alkaline and keto-friendly foods, without being too strict on themselves. The best part? As you start to shift your diet and lifestyle, gradually, step-by-step, with no stress or overwhelm, taking care of your nutrition and giving your body what it needs to stay healthy, all your bad habits and unwanted food cravings will be eventually going away. It's as simple as that.

So, don't be afraid to get started now, today! Forget about the whole "Oh, I need to be ready" thing. You are getting ready by shifting your mindset as you are going through a pretty long intro to this book! (it has a profound purpose and intention though).

Disclaimer:
I am not a medical doctor, and this book is not intended as a substitute for professional advice from your physician. To change your lifestyle successfully and healthily, I highly recommend regular check-ups, blood tests, and consultations with your physician.

This book is written as a simple inspirational guide to help you lose weight by eating a healthy, balanced diet. Sometimes, the "side effect" of a healthy weight loss diet (and losing weight in general) is that your other health issues may start to heal (it happened to a lot of my readers and friends). However, please note that the only goal of this book is weight loss, a positive mindset, and healthy recipes. An ethical framework is critical to me. While, now and then, I share the encouraging results that other people had on the alkaline keto lifestyle, I am by no way implying you will get the same results. To lose weight successfully and permanently, you must stay committed to the process of changing your lifestyle, one step at a time.

Also, if you are on medication or recovering from any disease, pregnant, lactating, or after surgery, I highly recommend you talk to your physician before changing your diet.

How Not to (Keto) Diet

I believe you can learn a lot from my early dieting mistakes, and they can save you a ton of time.

I will keep it short and sweet, though. I am sure you are already waiting for the 3 weight loss pillars and the new details of an alkaline keto lifestyle.

So, I started my weight loss journey with all kinds of crazy and restrictive fad diets. Counting calories (and reducing them massively). Going hungry. Zoning. You name it. I have tried it all! Only to end up feeling sick and tired and back to the same old, same old!

At the same time, as I was blindly experimenting with those fad diets, I would walk away from real foods. Instead, I was a big fan of processed shakes (low fat, of course), processed biscuits, and, of course, all the low-calorie stuff.

Little did I know that I was messing up my metabolism! Losing weight was hard. Even if I lost some weight here and there, I could never keep it off. I developed an identity of someone who could never lose weight no matter what, and so it was harder and harder to stay motivated.

I tried all kinds of low carb and high protein diets only to end up constipated and sluggish.

Things were getting more complicated as I was getting older. Back in the day, I could lose weight by over-exercising. But then, I got very sick, and so I began looking for healthier and whole food options.

The first thing I came across was a Paleo diet, and I am very grateful for it because it helped me transition to a more gluten-free and lactose-free lifestyle, which helped me heal my body. I began eating simple meals like fish or meat with some veggies, and I stopped eating fast food.

I did feel better on Paleo, but I still could not lose weight. So, I came across the vegan diet, and, since I have never been a meat person, really, it appealed to me a lot. I felt like going vegan because everyone was talking about it, and it seemed like the healthiest option on the planet.

And it made sense to me. I thought: *It's probably meat and eggs that were making me fat!*

I already quit dairy on a paleo diet, so it seemed like the next logical step to give this vegan thing a try. I have read lots of books written by vegan doctors, and I have also watched a lot of documentaries that eventually made me go vegan. I did my best to be a healthy vegan, and I focused on a whole food, low fat, plant-based vegan diet as it was advertised as the holy grail of everything.

It felt very good at first, and I began losing some weight. I was also happy as I thought I was a part of something bigger. Unfortunately, I felt weaker and weaker and eventually developed anemia. At first, it was just an iron-deficiency. I began taking supplements prescribed by my doctor. They didn't do much, unfortunately, and I was advised to add some animal products to my diet.

Eventually, I began researching online and found out there are a lot of people who just could not do a vegan plant-based diet.

Please note, I am not bashing a vegan diet, there are many people who do well on it and stay on it for many reasons. I am happy for them! But, since I am sharing my story here- it did not work for me. The good thing is that I got used to eating a lot of vegetables and making smoothies! And plants still form the vast majority of my diet!

The bad thing? Well, while on a vegan diet, I ate way too much fruit and drunk way too much fruit juice, therefore, increasing my sugar intake without even realizing it. I was always hungry, and I felt like snacking!

So then what happened it that I discovered an alkaline diet (will be diving more into it later) as Tony Robbins was talking about it in one of his seminars. It made sense to me because it seemed like a clean food diet, mostly plant-based (but without too much sugary fruit). It also allowed some quality animal products here and there if needed. I went for it, and I loved it!

The alkaline diet helped me heal my body and create a balance I wanted! Finally, I could eat lots of veggies, greens, and low-sugar fruit, as well as nuts and seeds, combined with some quality animal products whenever my body asked for them. It just seemed the perfect diet for me! I felt great, and I began losing weight. No more anemia, no more feeling sick all the time. Oh, and I also developed a massive passion for drinking green juices.

But...the real breakthrough came when I discovered the keto diet and combined it with the alkaline way of eating through the alkaline ketogenic lifestyle – precisely what I am sharing in this book!

Then I asked myself: *What if someone could just shorten the learning and experimentation curve and just dive right into the alkaline keto lifestyle to lose weight? Without having to repeat all my diet mistakes?*

Some of my readers and friends lost more weight in a month (using the alkaline ketogenic lifestyle) than they previously did in an entire decade! It's all about having the right information to follow! Now it's time for you to lose weight. For good! Before we dive into the weight loss pillars, let's do some accountability!

Email me at:
info@yourwellnessbooks.com and let me know what your weight loss goal is. It will help you stay committed and motivated!

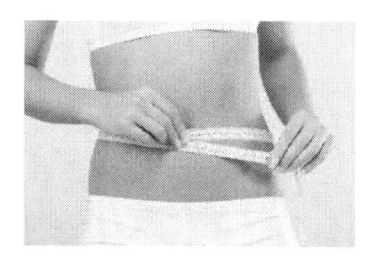

The 3 Missing Factors to Permanent and Healthy Weight Loss

It's time to make our weight loss pillars work for you!

Pillar #1 Use Good Fats to Lose Weight (aka the Keto Secret Paradox)

Imagine how good it would feel to be able to eliminate your carb and sugar cravings by giving your body what it needs to stop craving them! So that you no longer need to depend on will power and discipline to say no to processed sugar and carbs.

This weight loss pillar will show you exactly how to do it by getting to the root of the problem.

The biggest problem most people face is: *how do I stop those annoying sugar and carb cravings?* I have been there too. And trust me, switching to low calorie and low fat will not cut it. Low calorie and low-fat products can only strengthen your sugar and carb cravings.

Also, imagine how good it would feel to lose weight sustainably? So that you no longer suffer from the "yoyo" effect?

Trying to lose weight and having nothing to show for is annoying as heck. But…losing weight only to put it back on later is even more annoying because it makes you question everything. You keep asking yourself: *Was it even worth it?*

It's like working hard to get a promotion, getting it and then losing it.

Well, the fastest way to a yoyo effect are the following:
-will power alone (please note, I am not saying that working on your will power and discipline is useless; however the problem of unwanted cravings needs to be addressed from the inside out- you need to know what to put in your body to help it stop the cravings, so the latest motivational program, may not fully cut it).

-diet shakes with reduced fats and calories – their effect is very short-term, and even if you can lose weight fast using them, your body will eventually start demanding you feed it well, which will make you put all the weight you lost back on (and after diet shakes "starvation period" even healthy balanced meals can make you fat)

-over-exercising and feeling exhausted and probably stressed-out too (because all your free time when you are not working, or sleeping is spent working out - I mean, nobody can take it for a long time!).

-eating lettuce or overdoing all kinds of crazy detoxes or unrealistic cleanses – I am all for cleanses, but only well-designed, nutritionally balanced healthy, clean food cleanses. Good cleanses do not restrict your daily calorie intake. Instead, they focus on the quality of your calories and the foods that can help you lose weight and burn fat by stimulating your metabolism. *(if you are interested in cleansing, be sure to check out our recommended resources at the end of this book).*

So, here's the first thing you need to let go off to lose weight for good and feel amazing:
Don't be afraid of good fats! They will not make you fat!

All you need is to allow your body to tap into its own fat stores by switching your primary fuel source from carbs to fats.

This little switch alone will help you improve your health and balance your blood sugar.

You can go all in and become a hardcore keto-terian if you wish too. But, you can also make a simple, intuitive switch by reducing your intake of carbs and sugars while increasing your intake of good, healthy fats.

This is what this book is all about. We are not getting into complicated keto diets and micro-managing all our macros.
As I said before, there is nothing wrong with that, and it can serve its purpose, but it's not required to succeed on this lifestyle; an intuitive, flexible, but well-defined approach will suffice.

From my experience – most women (my primary reading audience) love simple, intuitive approaches to pretty much anything. At the same time, men prefer to get into details, count everything, etc. Whatever you prefer, be my guest, there is no right or wrong. But, once again, this is a simple-to-follow weight loss book, and if you want to lose weight and focus on what matters (taking consistent action), the simpler it gets, the better! And our intuitive approach will suffice.

A healthy, sustainable, and relatively fast weight loss all comes down to the right strategy that forms part of a well-defined system.

The GENERAL RULE is: Less carbs and more fats.
Surprisingly enough, by enriching your diet with more good fats, you will automatically crave less carbs and sugars!

Most diets take the "cut down on everything today" approach, and this is hard to follow, especially if you don't feed your body with foods (and drinks) that will make it crave less of the bad stuff. Saturated fats are not bad for you and will help you lose weight, think clearly, crave less sugar and carbs, and feel amazing. Our ancestors did not thrive on sugars or carbs. They did not have bagels, croissants, or processed bread. They used good, natural fats to keep going!

(If you want to dive deeper into learning more about the benefits of saturated fats, you may want to check out the book *The Big Fat Surprise* by Nina Teicholz).

The bad fats you want to avoid (please implement this as fast as possible) are industrially processed oils, for example, canola oil, processed margarine and processed vegetable oils (you will find full printable food lists at the end of this book).

You may also download them now by going to:

www.YourWellnessBooks.com/alkalineketo

Instead, focus on good fats:
Examples of Healthy Keto Fats & Oils
- Extra-virgin coconut oil
- Extra virgin olive oil (not for cooking, but great for salads and some veggie smoothies)
- Raw butter or ghee
- Grass-fed pasteurized butter or ghee
- Beef tallow
- Avocado and avocado oil
- organic bacon and meats
- fish and fish oil

Dietary fat does not equal body fat. The main culprit that makes you fat (and controls you and your mood) is sugar.

The fastest way to eliminate your sugar and carb cravings is by enriching your diet with good fats.

Here are some ideas, tips, and recipes you can start incorporating into your diet right now to begin transitioning to a healthy, weight loss stimulating lifestyle as fast as possible!

Coconut Oil Tips & Recipes to Eliminate Sugar Cravings

Whenever you crave sugar, have a tablespoon of coconut oil instead – these were the words of one of my alkaline nutrition teachers, and to be honest, I was very skeptical at first!

But then I tried it, and boy did it work! I even keep a jar of coconut oil at work, to "oil myself up" whenever needed!

Coconut Oil Cortado Style Coffee Recipe

This recipe is perfect if you are not a breakfast person!
Ingredients:
- 1 expresso
- 1 tablespoon coconut oil
- 2 tablespoons coconut milk

Instructions:
1. Combine all the ingredients in a small coffee cup.
2. Mix well, drink, and enjoy!

Creamy Cinnamon Latte Recipe

Cinnamon makes this coffee taste so nice, and it also prevents sugar cravings- we always want to tackle the problem from different angles!

Ingredients:
- 1 cup coconut milk, warm
- 1 expresso
- 2 tablespoons coconut oil
- 1 teaspoon cinnamon

Stevia to sweeten, if needed (it's a natural ingredient, it's not processed, and it has no sugar in it- the perfect addition to your drinks and smoothies if you like it sweet).

Instructions:
1. Blend all the ingredients in a hand blender.
2. Shake well, serve, and enjoy!

Green Tea Weight Loss Drink

This simple tea-based drink is perfect as a quick afternoon pick me up!

Ingredients:
- 1 cup of green tea
- 1 cup coconut milk
- 2 tablespoons coconut oil
- Stevia to sweeten if needed

Instructions:
Blend all the ingredients, serve, and enjoy!

Creamy Coconut Ice Cream Recipe

This one is perfect for hot summers!

Ingredients:
- 1 big avocado
- Half lime, peeled
- 1 cup thick coconut milk
- 2 tablespoons coconut oil
- 1 teaspoon cinnamon powder
- 1 teaspoon vanilla powder
- 10 drops of liquid stevia

Instructions:
1. Blend and freeze for a few hours (you can re-cycle an old ice cream container).
2. Enjoy! Yes, you can enjoy this ice cream to your heart's content!

Oh, and it doesn't have to be about coconut oil and coconut products. I get that some people may be allergic to coconut. You can also experiment with avocados and avocado oil as well as delicious creamy nut milk (such as almonds and cashews).

While you will find more recipes and simple meal plans at the end of this book, for now, let's have a look at some simple snack ideas filled with good fats so that you no longer crave sugar!

More Simple Recipes to Feed Your Body with Some Good Fats!

Spicy Avocado Smoothie

I love this smoothie whenever I feel like snacking...it satisfies my need for salt (salt can be healthy, and this is what we will be diving in the next weight loss pillar dedicated to alkaline diet and foods) as well as for something spicy.

Ingredients:
- 2 small avocados, peeled and pitted
- 1 cup almond or cashew milk, unsweetened and with no processed industrial oils in it
- Pinch of chili powder or a mini chili flake
- Pinch of Himalayan salt
- 1 tablespoon extra-virgin olive oil

Instructions:
Blend all the ingredients in a blender, serve and enjoy!

Anti-Stress Infusion

This delicious tea is just perfect for helping you unwind and sleep better while eliminating sugar cravings.

Ingredients:
- 1 cup Melissa tea
- Half cup coconut or almond milk (unsweetened)
- 1 tablespoon coconut oil

Instructions:
1. Combine all the ingredients, serve, and enjoy!

Cashew Nut Crew Snacks

If you can't stop snacking – don't worry. Instead of snacking on sugar and carbs, try these keto style fat bombs!

Ingredients:
- Half cup cashews
- Half cup almonds
- 4 tablespoons coconut oil
- A few drops of stevia, if needed
- Cinnamon powder

Instructions:
1. Blend the nuts and coconut, adding a bit of stevia if you want.
2. Form little bombs and sprinkle some cinnamon powder on top.
3. Serve and enjoy!

So, these were a few simple snacks and drink ideas to help you drastically reduce your cravings for sugar and carbs by adding in some good fats.

Below, you will find a few more simple recipes and meal ideas, you can start implementing today or tomorrow, even before you are done reading this book. You will find more recipes and meal guidance at the end of this book, but I just couldn't help myself, and I really wanted to give you some recipe ideas now so that you could get started as you are reading this book (FYI, some people start losing weight without even reading this entire program!).

Egg Butter Avocado Breakfast or Brunch

Ingredients:
- 2 or 3 organic eggs
- 2 tablespoons grass-fed butter
- 1 avocado, peeled and pitted
- Himalayan salt, black pepper and Italian spices to season

Instructions:
1. Fry the eggs in butter.
2. When ready, serve with the avocado and season with spices and salt.
3. Enjoy!

The 5 Ingredient 5 Minute Salad

Ingredients:
- 3 big slices of smoked salmon, cut into smaller pieces
- 2 big tomatoes, sliced
- 1 big cucumber, peeled and sliced
- Italian spices and salt
- Olive or avocado oil

Instructions:
1. Combine all the ingredients in a salad bowl.
2. Toss well, serve and enjoy!

Easy Mediterranean Tuna Salad

Ingredients:
- 2 cans of tuna
- Half cup black or green olives, pitted
- A few slices of goat cheese
- A few onion rings
- 1 cup arugula leaves
- 1 tablespoon apple cider vinegar
- 2 tablespoons avocado or olive oil
- Himalayan salt and Italian spices to season

Instructions:
1. Combine all the ingredients in a salad bowl.
2. Serve and enjoy!

For now, all you need to notice is this – we are focusing on good fats, veggies (naturally low in sugar), and some quality animal products. This way of eating is simple, and the meals are very easy to prepare.

There is a lot of controversy behind the keto diet, as it basically turned the standard food pyramid upside down, and it stays away from processed sugars and crappy carbs that our society can't live without!

But, when you have a look at our simple and balanced meals and ingredient combinations, it's actually a very simple approach to healthy eating- something that our ancestors would thrive on.

They did not have access to processed carbs and sugar, nor did they have access to brainwashing media channels and fear-based marketing that, very often, tells us the exact opposite of what we should be doing.

Everyone is different, and there is no one size fits all diet. Hence, I am a big believer in an intuitive and flexible (without overindulging though) approach. Take small baby steps to start experimenting with the tips and recipes from this book. Listen to your body and be kind to yourself!

The keto approach is all about focusing on low carb, high fat, and moderate protein so that your body can start using fat for fuel (a state of the so-called: ketosis).

The ketogenic diet goes way beyond weight loss programs as it has also been used in clinical settings to heal epilepsy and diabetes (the keto diet is naturally very low in sugar and usually recommended for diabetics or pre-diabetics).

Keto works as true fasting as it detoxes, restores, and replenishes your body. It also produces healthy mitochondria (healthy cells to help you enjoy more energy).

Imagine how your life would change if only you could enjoy more energy naturally? Without having to rely on coffee all the time? Before discovering keto, I was a caffeine addict, and even with all the coffee, I drank I felt lethargic. My body got used to it, and I felt even more tired. But after I switched to the alkaline ketogenic lifestyle, my energy levels skyrocketed. Yes, I still like to enjoy more morning coffee with some coconut oil in it. Some people use butter. I just don't like butter in my coffee. Still, you could give it a go, it's keto!

With more energy, you get more happiness and motivation. Suddenly pursuing your goals is fun! This is what this lifestyle can do for you; it's not only about weight loss (although right now, I get it- you want to start losing weight).

On another note, more energy can lead you to suddenly wanting exercise more so that you can tone your body and get rid of toxins at the same time. Abundant energy can change your life!

Think about that promotion you have always wanted to get. Or maybe you want to start a side hustle, passion project, or do some extra hours at work to earn more money. Well, with more energy, everything is possible, doable and more fun!

This is exactly what happens when you eat less carbs and sugars while adding more good fats into your diet. The good news- you can achieve it even without going ultra-hardcore keto (nothing wrong with that, BTW, do whatever works for you).

Remember when I mentioned my alkaline nutrition teacher who told me: *Whenever you crave sugar or carbs, have a generous tablespoon of coconut oil instead*?

At that time, I had no idea about the keto lifestyle, but that tip alone, alongside adding more avocados and fish oil into my diet, was a real game-changer for me.

A friend of mine (she is a hardcore "ketoterian") says that there are only 2 diets. The keto diet is one of them. The second diet is anything that is not keto or doesn't use good fats as fuel.

I am not that extreme, so I like to say there are 3 kinds of diets. The first one is the Standard Western Diet (Or Standard American Diet- aka the SAD diet) consisting of fast food and processed foods with the nasty chemicals in them. Then, there is a clean food diet – anything that uses real foods (it is already a fantastic step forward!).

Just getting rid of fast and processed foods as well as soda and fizzy sugary drinks is an excellent move for most people!). Finally, the third diet (actually more of a lifestyle than a diet) is the alkaline keto way of eating- which is a clean food diet that is cleverly optimized to help you burn fat and lose weight almost on autopilot, by giving your body exactly what it needs to lose weight.

Keto is the most effective approach to help you burn fat, and it helps you use fat as a primary energy source while ridding your system out of sugars (and the need to crave them and consume them all the time).

The exciting thing is that as soon as you start shifting to an alkaline keto lifestyle, your taste buds will change and you will no longer enjoy foods or drinks with an excessive amount of sugar. It will no longer be who you are and what you want.

It will feel natural for you, and you will no longer have to rely on your will power and discipline alone.

Eating fats and restricting carbs (to 25 g net -which is total carbs minus fiber-a day) puts you in nutritional ketosis.

(If you would like to dive deeper into this, I highly recommend you take this free keto test to get your personalized keto plan: www.YourWellnessBooks.com/keto)

However, as I said before, this is not necessary. As long as you get rid of, or drastically reduce processed carbs (pasta, bread, rice) as well as sugar and sugary fruit such as bananas and you add more good fats into your diet- you are good to go. With such an approach, you don't need to worry about counting everything unless you want to.

Your body can only become an excellent fat burner and fat adapter when it's fed fats, and it's not reliant on carbs.

Most people who transition their diet in a more ketogenic direction while letting go of processed carbs and fast food, say: Wow, Finally, I have more energy! Finally, I can work better and faster, and I got that promotion. Suddenly, I can fit into those jeans that were waiting for me for years.

At the same time, the keto lifestyle acts as a natural anti-inflammatory diet, and it can also improve your gut health. All in a simple, natural way by helping us get back to our roots and eat foods that are good for us!

The First Weight Loss Pillar in a Nutshell…

To sum up the first pillar and the keto paradox (consume more fats to turn your body into a fat-burning machine, as it was naturally designed to):

By reducing carbs and adding more good fats into your diet, you have the power to lose weight, burn fat, while enjoying steady mood and energy.

You can finally give yourself the freedom to STOP thinking about the food and snacks all the time! Your blood sugar will stabilize, and you will no longer feel bloated.

Oh…but Elena! Are you telling me that keto isn't restrictive? I like my pasta and pizza.

OK, so this time, there is no good news and bad news. There is good news and good news!

Good news #1 You can still enjoy your favorite foods now and then, for example, on a family occasion or during weekends or special events. It's not that you will never be able to eat pizza again! At the same time, your favorite foods can be made in a healthier, more alkaline-ketogenic friendly version. For example, you could go for a gluten-free and low carb pizza while adding natural and whole foods on top (therefore avoiding nasty chemicals, fast food, and other nasty stuff).

Or you could make a nice zucchini pizza with some fresh cheese and home-made pesto.

Not an ultra keto meal (for all those fastidious readers who fear every mini microgram of carbs). But hey! It's packed with nutrients, good fats, is healthy and unprocessed.

And yes, I will be the first one to admit that I like to indulge in my favorite foods once in a while, especially during family occasions or when we go out during the weekend. However, I take care of my diet during the week. Whenever I go out for a meal, I optimize what I eat and drink before and after so that I can create balance and allow my body to process the overindulgence as fast and smoothly as possible.

Also, on the weekends, I move my body and work out more (walking and swimming), so I feel like I keep the balance. It works well for me!

Now, good news #2
When you experience the benefits of the alkaline keto lifestyle, your unhealthy food cravings will stabilize. So, the meals and foods you used to find the pleasure in will be no longer so tempting. As soon as you get to the alkaline keto side, you will no longer look back! You will burn all the bridges!

The real freedom is when you are in charge of what you eat, and you choose your foods, they don't choose you! It feels great and very empowering too.

By adding more fats into your diet and reducing carbs and sugars, you will be able to experience the real diet freedom while stabilizing your mood and food cravings. You will even find yourself with more free time!

I used to be a smoker, and before I committed to quitting, I used to think: *Oh, do I want to quit? I will lose my freedom; I will no longer be able to socialize with my co-workers or going out for a cigarette break.*

However, after quitting smoking, my way of thinking shifted. I can now experience true freedom by not smoking (aside from that, I can save money too, smoking can be an expensive habit!). Now, I use my breaks for meditation or journaling, and other people got inspired by my transformation.

So….don't look for excuses before you have tried it!

Oh, and the good news #3 is – the smoking example I used is a bit hardcore. However, when it comes to your diet- just try to follow the alkaline keto lifestyle most of the time and allow yourself a few exceptions on special occasions. I am a big fan of developing a healthy relationship with food. Life can already be complicated and stressful enough.
So…your diet should be as simple and easy as possible, and stress-free too!

I can still remember what it was like reading all those nutrition and diet books. Most of them were just so serious! And most of the writers and publishers behind them used holier than though attitudes that would just make me feel bad about myself.
Well! Not here, my friend, not here!

Now, it's time to dive into our Second Weight Loss Pillar that will help you maximize your weight loss success!

Weight Loss Pillar #2 Alkaline Autopilot for Smooth Weight Loss and Effortless Keto Lifestyle

In this book, we are learning how to attack excess weight and fat from all the angles possible. And aside from using keto-friendly fats, we also need to use what I like to call the Alkaline Autopilot!
You see, to burn fat and lose weight effectively, your body needs certain micronutrients as well as alkaline electrolytes.

Many people go keto, but they have no idea about alkaline foods or drinks and end up feeling depleted of energy and eventually give up.

Below is the email I got from one of our readers after I had released the *Alkaline Ketogenic Mix* book (the first book in our *Alkaline Keto* series):

"Hi Elena,
I just breezed through your book The Alkaline Ketogenic Mix and wow great stuff! Recently I have been reading about alkaline keto lifestyle plans on some thyroid blogs I follow. I don't know how I haven't ever heard about this before now I'm just astounded!
(...)I have been doing a ketogenic diet for close to a year now with no real, sustainable results. I'm looking forward to implementing the alkaline foods for not only more variety but also to rid the acidity in my body. Prior to that I did paleo for years and healed my body from getting off gluten and dairy.
Well, thank you for the great information, and I look forward to hearing from you. "

You see, keto works when done correctly in a healthy and balanced way (that also includes alkaline foods). However, most people dive into keto by taking the main-stream approach, which consists of living on bacon, some eggs, butter, fat meats with no greens or veggies at all. OK, I know I am exaggerating here, but it's just to give you the overall picture.

If you want to stay healthy and live a real, balanced, alkaline keto lifestyle, you need to master the art of combining nutrient and mineral-rich alkaline foods (such as veggies and healthy greens) with keto foods and quality animal products.

Some people (like me, for example) will lean more towards the plant-based side (I have never been a big meat lover); some people, on the other hand, will lean more towards the animal-product side. However, in both cases, alkaline balance is needed.

This section will teach you everything you need to know about alkaline foods and drinks and how to combine them with keto for optimal results.

The Most Common Keto Mistakes

Overdoing animal products without providing your body with enough alkaline foods and alkaline minerals can lead to very unpleasant "keto detox" symptoms, which make it hard for most people to keep going.

The mainstream keto diet lacks fiber and minerals. Most people learn that fruit is rich in carbs, and since they want to go ultra keto, they fear it and let go of it. The good news is that there are different kinds of fruits, and there are many fruits you should incorporate into your alkaline keto lifestyle for optimal balance.

Keto is much easier and more effective with alkaline foods. At the same time, the alkaline diet is much more effective (and easier) with some quality animal products.

(I have done a hardcore vegan diet before, and it didn't work for me; however alkaline diet is not the same as the vegan diet and can be combined with quality animal products).

Strict keto diets can lead you to crash and burn. Once again, it's hard to do if your only weapon is will power. However, combining keto with alkaline is so much easier.

The reason why this is the second step is to make it easier for my readers. Most people fear veggies and greens and might find it easier to get started just by learning more about good fats and incorporating them into their diets.

However, we want to keep it as effective as possible!

I get many emails from my readers who go through my *Alkaline Keto* book series and tell me: *Wow, I finally get it, now I feel like I can do keto and live a healthy balanced, energized lifestyle!*
So, what exactly do you need to add our Alkaline Autopilot into your secret weight loss and fat burn weapons?

The Alkaline Lesson #1 – You Need Alkaline Minerals

There is no way around it; you just need them. Every day. Especially if you want to stay vibrant and full of energy.

Alkaline minerals include:
-calcium
-potassium
-magnesium
-sodium

Most people get enough calcium, but not enough potassium and sodium. And, most people are magnesium deficient. Yes, some supplements (if prescribed by your doctor) can help, but if your body is out of balance, it may be hard to absorb them.

A natural, clean food approach is the best long-term remedy!

The first thing you can start implementing is to use Himalayan salt. I use it for all my meals, and sometimes I like to add it to my water. *Lemon water, to be specific, lemons are also very rich in alkaline minerals. They are naturally low sugar fruits, which makes them both keto and alkaline-friendly – more on that later, in the food lists section!*

At the same time, you want to start adding more greens to your diet, for example:
-spinach
-kale
-arugula
-basil
-parsley
-cilantro

These can be sneaked into your smoothies.

Here is my alkaline-keto friendly, low-carb and low-sugar smoothie template:

- 1 avocado, peeled and pitted
- 1 cup coconut or nut milk
- 1 teaspoon chia seeds
- A few lime slices (you can also use lemons or grapefruits)
- A handful of greens of your choice
- 1 teaspoon coconut oil
- A pinch of Himalayan salt

Blend well, serve, and enjoy!

But for now, let's have a look at this simple **Soup-Style Smoothie Recipe Template:**

-1 avocado, peeled and pitted
-half cup veggies of your choice (for example steamed zucchini or broccoli, or raw red bell pepper)
-half cup greens of your choice
-1-2 tomatoes
-1 tablespoon oil (for example avocado or extra virgin olive oil)
-a few onion rings or 1 garlic clove
-a bit of water and plant-based milk or nut milk (almond or coconut milk or cashew milk)
-Himalayan salt and spices to season

Blend all the ingredients into a smoothie.
Serve as a raw soup and add in some hard-boiled eggs or meat leftovers to enjoy a quick, nutrient-packed meal!

The bottom line is – don't fear greens. Even if you hate kale or spinach, you can try greens such as arugula, cilantro, or basil and use them for your smoothies. If you have a juicer, you can also start juicing your greens. Yes, there is a way to make alkaline-keto friendly juices. All you need to do is to focus on low sugar ingredients, such as:

-greens

-veggies

-low sugar fruits such as limes, lemons, and grapefruits

You can spice up your juices with some Himalayan salt and olive oil, or plant-based milk. I usually juice every day or every other day, typically in the late afternoon. It helps me stay energized, and ever since I got on the green juice wagon, I feel more focused! It works great for me! During weekends I juice more, and I usually make a fresh juice every Saturday or Sunday morning.

While juicing is a bit more advanced and requires more preparation, smoothies are faster and easier for most people. So, if you are wondering where to start – go for smoothies for now. But, be sure to give juicing a try at some point!

For now, let's have a look at some simple, alkaline-friendly tweaks you can implement right away:

Tip #1 Drink filtered water with some lemon or lime and Himalayan salt to take care of your electrolyte balance

You can get alkaline water filters very inexpensively from Amazon, and they will help you save a ton of money on bottled water (which is not a healthy option).

Tip #2 Snack on avocados with some lemon juice and Himalayan salt. You can also add in some herbs, chopped tomatoes, and olive oil if you want.

Tip #3 Drink fresh tomato juice or smoothies- tomatoes are very rich in alkaline minerals, vitamin C, and other alkaline micronutrients you need for optimal balance. At the same time, they are very low in sugar and rich in beta-carotene to help you have healthy-looking, glowing skin.

Here's my homemade tomato juice recipe:
Ingredients:
-5 big tomatoes, peel removed
-1 cup water, filtered, preferably alkaline
-half cup coconut or almond milk
-1 teaspoon Italian spices
-a generous pinch of Himalayan salt
-black pepper if needed
-1 tablespoon olive oil

Blend and enjoy!

Tip #4 Snack on nuts and seeds such as almonds, add them to your smoothies and salads

Tip #5 Drink coconut water -it's naturally sweet, alkaline-friendly and jam-packed with healthy alkaline minerals, such as Magnesium

Tip #6 Serve your keto meals with big, green salads and always balance out animal products, such as meat, fish, or eggs with greens and veggies.

To sum up -no alkaline foods in your diet will lead to a bad and very ineffective (or short-term) keto experience filled with keto flu and fatigue.

However, alkaline foods will help you optimize your healthy eating plan while helping you stay more energized and motivated.
I have already mentioned that most people are Magnesium deficient (I highly recommend you do blood tests to see if you are one of them), and they also lack other alkaline minerals.
So, as far as other minerals are concerned...

According to the American Heart Association, you need about 2300 mg of sodium a day (it can be more if you live in a hot climate, or are an athlete). That's 1-2 teaspoons of Himalayan salt a day (I like to add a pinch to my water too!). Some alkaline nutritionists and experts recommend as much as 3000mg of sodium (or more) per day.

As for other alkaline minerals, you need:
Potassium- about 3500-4700 mg a day
Magnesium – 400-500 mg a day
Calcium – 1110 mg a day

Adding more healthy greens into your diet will help you increase your intake of these vital minerals.
Also, if you find it hard to sleep, your heart is pounding, and you are feeling stressed, chances are you are Magnesium deficient.

OK, so now, let's dive deeper into alkaline foods as well as their ability to help you burn fat and lose weight!

Understanding the Alkaline Diet to Lose Weight and Keep It Off

Going green is the best way to describe an alkaline lifestyle because the focus is on green vegetables in general, as they are the most alkaline food you can ingest. By ingesting alkaline foods and beverages, you can nourish and detox your entire system, causing it to function at its best. The benefits of the alkaline diet are numerous. Let us name a few:

Natural and Sustainable Weight Loss
-An alkaline diet will assist you in losing weight. One way that it does this is obvious. All of the foods you will be eating are very healthy, rich in minerals, and other healthy nutrients to help your body feel nourished (when your body feels nourished, it doesn't crave unhealthy foods).
-You will also be reducing the amount of acid in your body. The body stores fat to protect itself from an abundance of acid. It is a self-preservation method. This is part of the reason why people who eat a Standard Western diet can't lose weight, even if they restrict calories. Their bodies are clinging to that fat to minimize the effects of all of the acid in their systems.
-Another benefit of an alkaline lifestyle regarding weight loss is that alkaline systems have more oxygen in their cells. Oxygen is an essential part of eliminating fat cells from the body. The more oxygen in your system, the more efficient your metabolism will be.

Energy, Improved Mood and Increased Motivation on the Alkaline Diet
Going green does not only give you energy for the apparent reason that you are eating many more healthy, energizing vitamins. You

are negating the acid-induced lethargy that is brought on by an unhealthy acid-forming diet.

Not only do our bodies need an abundance of oxygen to lose weight, but we also need oxygen in our cells to energize us. The lack of oxygen in our cells causes fatigue. No, it is not just because you worked too late or partied to hard the night before. It is internal. If your cells are trying to function in a highly acidic environment, they will not be able to transfer oxygen efficiently; leading of course to exhaustion.

Cells in the body also make something that is called adenosine triphosphate (ATP). If your system is very acidic, it has an adverse effect on the ability of your cells to produce it. In the scientific world, it is known as the "energy currency of life." The ATP molecule contains the energy that we need to accomplish most things that we do (both internally and externally).

Increased Health, Balance, and Vitality

Another benefit of the alkaline lifestyle is that your body will be able to function at an optimum level instead of being inhibited by acids:

- Your heartbeat is thrown off by acidic wastes in the body. The stomach suffers greatly from over-acidity.
- The liver's job is to get rid of acid toxins, but also to produce alkaline enzymes. By simply reducing your acid intake, you can internally boost your alkalinity thanks to your liver!
- The lymph fluids function most efficiently in an alkaline system. They remove acid waste. Acidic systems not only have a slower lymph flow causing acids to be stored; they

can also cause acids to be reabsorbed through lymphatic ducts in your intestines that would typically be excreted.

Mental Focus on the Alkaline Diet

Just as the rest of the body is poorly affected by acid-forming foods and other toxins, so is your brain. And as we all know, it should be possible to control your emotions and decision making with your mind. Guess what? If your body is too acidic and is not alkaline, your mental clarity will be cloudy; your decision making could be off, as well as your emotional state.

Detox

Another huge benefit of an alkaline lifestyle is detoxification. First, you are going to be cutting out foods that are continually adding toxins to your system. Secondly, you are going to be eating foods that allow your body to detox and rid itself of the acids that have built up in your system all this time. When we detoxify our bodies, our emotions, bodily functions, and mental functions are able to operate at their optimum levels.

Here's one thing to understand- the hardcore keto (or even paleo diet) that is focused mostly on animal products can be very acid-forming to your body.

Your body can then start to store fat as a natural protection to counterbalance the acids.

By incorporating more alkaline foods into your diet (and combining them with a balanced keto approach), not only will you lose weight, but you will also create an incredibly healthy lifestyle you love!

Going Alkaline in an Easy Way

Alkaline vs. Acidic? Sounds like the title fight for a light-weight boxing match. In reality, it is a fight, a fight for the pH balance of your body. pH levels are the measure of how acidic a liquid is. Our bodies function optimally when our blood is at about 7.365 ph. pH levels range from 0 to 14. 0 is the highest level of acidity, but basically everything 0-7 would be considered acidic. The 7-14 range is alkaline.

It's NOT about RAISING or changing your pH
I very often get emails from brainwashed readers. I mean, I did not influence them; they are coming from other books or blogs. My goal is to give people the honest truth and well-researched information with no hype.

So, back to people who email me. They somehow got this idea that there are some secret superfoods or supplements that will raise their pH, and as soon as their pH is raised, they will cure all of their diseases and lose weight overnight. However, it doesn't work that way.

And, as someone very passionate about alkaline foods, I will be the first one to admit that even though it's a very useful tool, it's not an overnight cure or some magic solution to make all your problems go away.

There is lots of misinformation out there, and so the alkaline diet gets lots of bad rep. Therefore, many people call it some quackery pseudoscience. Skeptics say – *how can this diet work if you can't change your body pH? Your stomach's pH is acidic anyway, so what's the point?*

And yes, they are right. You can't change or raise your body's pH. Also, the alkaline diet is not about changing or altering your stomach's pH, which is and should stay acidic.

The alkaline <u>diet is not about changing or "raising" your pH</u>. This is where many alkaline guides go wrong. You see, our body is smart enough to self-regulate our pH for us, no matter what we eat.

Unfortunately, when you constantly bombard your body with acid-forming foods (for example, processed foods, fast food, alcohol, sugar, and even too much meat or animal products, you torture your body with incredible stress. Why? Well, because it has to work harder to maintain that optimal pH.

Here's a simple example.
Imagine you immerse yourself in a bath filled with ice. You say, but hey, my body can self-regulate its optimal temperature, right? And yes, it can. But it will eventually collapse, and you will get ill. The same happens with nutrition and our blood pH. You can spend years indulging in toxic, processed, acid-forming foods that only deprive your body of its vital nutrients, saying: "But hey, my body will self-regulate its optimal blood pH."

And again, it will. But sooner or later, it will give up and manifest a disease. It will accumulate fat as its natural defense function to protect your body from over-acidity. We don't want to end up there, right? Remember, **your body stores fat to protect itself from over-acidity.**

So, to sum up- the alkaline diet is a natural, holistic system, a nutritional lifestyle that advocates the consumption of fresh, unprocessed foods that are rich in nutrients. These are called alkaline foods, and they help your body stimulate its optimal healing functions. Yes! A healthy body needs nutrients, and fresh low sugar fruits and vegetables are great for that.

The problem is that nowadays, most diets are filled with acid-forming foods that eventually make it hard for the body to regulate its optimal, healthy blood pH, and artificial sweeteners do the same. Acidosis is very common in this day and age thanks to things we drink as well: caffeine and sugar drinks, alcohol, and sodas all have an acidic effect on our bodies. Not to mention the chemicals many people take in through things like smoking and drugs (even prescription drugs have this effect). Then, you go on another "diet", you reduce your calories and you over-exercise, yet you can't lose weight.

Well. Alkalinity is one of the missing factors here…

There are many ways that you could become acidic. Eating acid-forming foods, stress, taking in too many toxins, and bodily processes all-cause acidity in the body.

Our internal systems try to balance themselves out and bring pH up with the help of alkaline minerals that we can ingest through our diet. If we do not take in a higher percentage of alkaline than acidic foods, we can become too acidic.

When you are acidic, it makes every process that your body does typically much more difficult or impossible for it to accomplish (including weight loss).

We cannot absorb the beneficial nutrients we need from our food properly. Our cells are not able to produce energy efficiently. Our bodies are not able to fix damaged cells properly. We will not be able to detoxify properly. Fatigue and illness will drag you down.

Sounds horrible; does it not? Here are some signs that you are overly acidic:
-Feeling tired all the time. You have no physical or mental drive at all.
-You always feel cold.
-You get sick all the time.
-You are depressed or just feel "blah" all the time for no real reason (I had this problem and thought it was hormonal changes).
-You get headaches for no apparent reason
-You get watery eyes or inflamed eyelids.
-Your teeth are sensitive and may crack or chip
-Your gums are inflamed, and you are susceptible to canker sores (I, James, thought this was genetic, but now know better).
-Acidic stomach with acid indigestion and reflux can be an issue
-Your fingernails crack, split, and break
-You have super dry hair that sheds and is hay-like with split ends
-Your skin breaks out in acne or is irritated when you sweat
-You get leg cramps and spasms
-You get nervous and can't sleep. It's always a battle to get up!

If you feel acidic, one of the best things you could do is to go on an alkaline cleanse to help your body heal from over acidity. An alkaline cleanse program, is aimed at eating 100% alkaline, for a short period of time, to help your body release acidic toxins and restore your energy and balance.

You can find more information in the recommended resources section, and the end of this book.

An alkaline cleanse program will prepare your body for more amazing changes, including weight loss. Personally, I do an alkaline cleanse every year. Hey, it's only for a week or two and it can really help you reclaim your health!

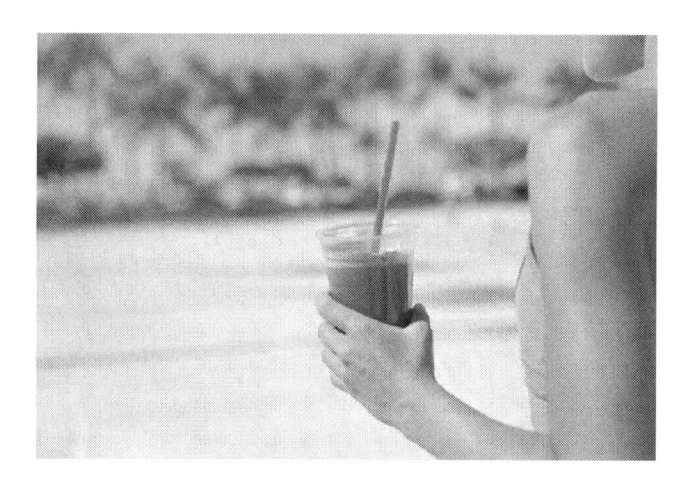

Is Alkaline Diet Hard to Follow?

Many people complain that the alkaline diet is hard to follow. But the way we see it is this- it's perfect! Plus, it's not a diet; it's a lifestyle.

You don't have to be 100% perfect. Simply make sure that MOST of your diet consist of quality alkaline foods, and the rest can be quality animal products. It's all about balance!

Unfortunately, most people don't even eat 5% alkaline...hence they end up feeling acidic and tired.

What are alkaline foods? Is it about their pH?

No, luckily, it's much, much easier. We don't care about the food's pH in its natural form. All we care about is the effect that the food has on the body after it has been consumed and metabolized. For example, lemons, grapefruits, and limes are considered alkaline-forming foods.

What? Elena? Are you out of your mind? Everyone knows lemons are acidic!

Well, let me repeat again. Lemons are acidic as far as their taste and ph. in their natural state are concerned. But, they are full of alkaline minerals and low in sugar, which makes them alkaline-forming foods.

At the same time, oranges contain more sugar, which makes them less alkaline-forming.

It's that simple!

As a general rule, alkaline foods are:
- rich in minerals and vitamins
- fresh, not packaged
- not fermented
- low in sugar (all kinds of sugar are acid-forming)
- plant-based
- mostly raw or slightly cooked
- caffeine-free
- chemical-free
- provide hydration

As a general rule, acid-forming foods are:
- full of chemicals
- low in nutrients
- high in sugar
- contain caffeine, alcohol, toxins
- processed
- packaged
- fermented
- contain artificial ingredients
- animal by-products

The reason why so many other charts show such disparity is because they base their classifications on the readings for the so-called PRAL, which stands for Potential Renal Acid Load research. Unfortunately, this is not a reliable source of practical information for us.

Why?

Well, PRAL tests burn the food at extreme temperature and then take a read of the 'ash' that is left behind and what it's pH is.

While this will give a read of its alkalinity from the mineral content of the food, by burning it at such a high temperature, they also burn away sugar. And sugar is very acid-forming...

That is why, on some charts, high sugar fruits are listed as super alkaline. However, high-sugar fruit such as bananas is not alkaline-forming to the body, and it's not keto either.

Some charts determine acidity or alkalinity on the food before it is consumed & others like the ones we list below are more interested in the effect the food has on the body after it has been consumed.

We have a simple to follow alkaline-acid food lists (printable) you can grab for free at:

www.yourwellnessbooks.com/charts

To sum up, what we have learned so far:

Pillar #0 – Commit to short daily exercise
Pillar #1 – Focus on good fats (and reduce carbs)
Pillar #2 – Eat more alkaline foods and drink more alkaline beverages (lemon water, smoothies, tomato juice, etc.)

Now, it's time to dive into the final weight loss pillar – putting it all together and taking imperfect massive action with delicious, flexible, and totally customizable meal plans and recipes!

Weight Loss Pillar #3 Right Food Lists, Right Mindset & Easy Recipes You Will Love!

Let's start off with alkaline keto food lists. The following information does all the heavy lifting for you!

You can also visit our private website at:
www.YourWellnessBooks.com/alkalineketo
to grab your food lists as a printable PDF (free of course) and use them whenever you go shopping.

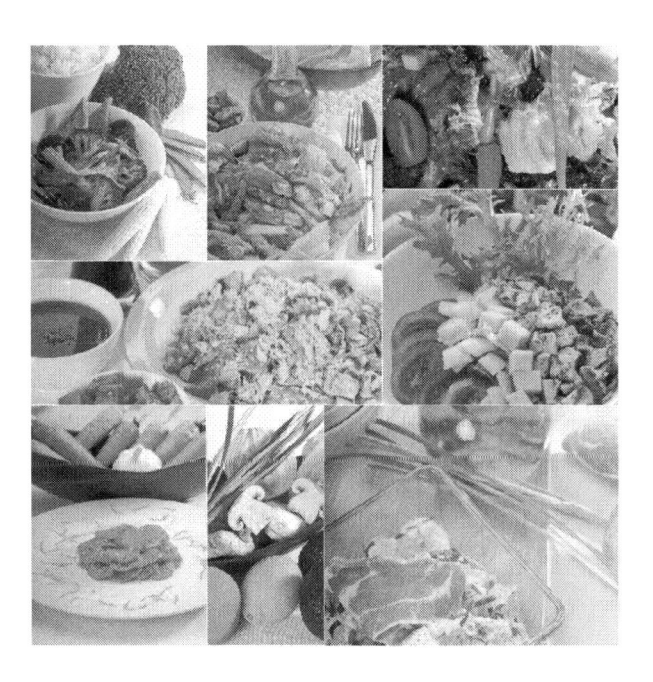

Alkaline Keto Food Lists & Recipes for Massive Weight Loss

Your alkaline-keto-friendly food lists

The following foods can be eaten to your heart's content!
Oh, and when it comes to eating meat, you can choose fattier cuts. In fact, you totally should!

When choosing fish, choose all wild-caught fish with fins and scales. Industrial fish is full of toxins and not good for you.

All kinds of veggies are excellent, and making sure you serve your keto meals on heaps of greens will help you stay fully nourished and prevent sugar cravings too.

Also, please note that the food lists below are designed for an average, busy person who simply wishes to stay healthy, energized, or lose some weight. So, they are a bit simplified. If you have any specific goals, whether it's athletic, or healing any particular health issue, I would recommend you invest in a dietician specializing in ketogenic diets and alkaline foods so that they can create personalized food lists for you and your desired outcome.

Keto - Meat (try to go for organic)
- Beef
- Lamb
- Turkey
- Duck
- Chicken
- Goat
- Venison
- Veal
- Buffalo
- Elk

- As well as **all organ meats such as liver, kidney, etc.** of above animals

Keto - Fish (try to go for freshly caught)
- Salmon
- Mackerel
- tuna
- haddock
- halibut
- bass
- trout
- sole
- herring
- snapper
- sardines
- whitefish
- whiting

+ as well as a roe from any of these fish
+All kinds of bone broths and stocks of above meat and fish are allowed
+ Dried and cured meats from the above-mentioned animals and fish are allowed

Keto - Eggs and Dairy Products
- organic free-range chicken eggs
- duck and goose organic free-range eggs
- raw full-fat cheeses
- raw cream
- all types of kefir - Raw or organic
- pasteurized cow's milk, goat's milk
- sheep's milk

Alkaline Keto Food Lists & Recipes for Massive Weight Loss

Please note- Dairy products can be skipped if you are lactose intolerant. Most recipes from this book use plant-based milk that is both alkaline and keto-friendly (coconut milk, almond milk, etc.). Personally, I am not a big fan of cow's milk (doesn't work well for me and my digestion and is also very acid-forming).

It's really up to you. I like to have a little bit of organic cheese or organic kefir every now and then. But, most of the time, I live a dairy-free lifestyle.

Alkaline Keto Veggies
- **All green leafy vegetables:**
- Spinach
- Kale
- swiss chard
- chicory
- romaine and iceberg lettuce
- little gem
- radicchio
- dandelion
- lettuce
- greens,
- chives
- lettuce
- bok choy
- mustard greens
- turnip greens
- nasturtium
- watercress,
- rocket/arugula

- Micro-greens seed sprouts
- Bell pepper

All cruciferous vegetables:
- broccoli
- cabbage
- radish
- kohlrabi
- horseradish
- daikon
- collard greens
- cauliflower
- brussels sprouts
- spring greens

Other non-starchy vegetables:
- artichoke
- asparagus
- avocado
- celery
- endive
- fennel
- garlic

Herbs
- Basil
- Cilantro
- Mint
- parsley

Other:
- kelp
- leeks
- okra
- olives
- onion
- spring/green onions
- water
- shallots
- mushrooms (not considered alkaline by most alkaline experts, however, can be added in small amounts and are still keto friendly).
- chestnuts

Alkaline Grasses
- wheatgrass juice
- barley grass juice

Healthy Keto Fats & Oils (the ones coming from plants are also alkaline)
- Extra-virgin coconut oil
- Extra virgin olive oil (not for cooking)
- Raw butter or ghee
- Grass-fed pasteurized butter or ghee
- Beef tallow
- Goat's milk butter (not for cooking)
- Coconut milk cream (organic, with no additives)
- Coconut butter

Condiments
- All kinds of organic spices, herbs, and pepper
- Unrefined sea salt, Himalaya salt, and rock salt
- Organic Mustard (with no artificial additives)
- Organic Apple cider vinegar
- Balsamic vinegar (with no artificial additives)
- Organic Mayonnaise (made with only natural oils, no vegetable oil)
- Fresh home-made guacamole

Keto Friendly Fermented Foods
- Raw, lacto-fermented sauerkraut
- Raw, lacto-fermented kimchi
- Dairy probiotic foods listed - such as kefir and raw milk products
- Pickled vegetables (must be raw, lactofermented)

Drinks
- Filtered water
- Alkaline water
- Herbal infusions (caffeine-free)
- Sparkling mineral water

- Bone broth
- Filtered water with fresh lemon or lime
- Green juice with no high sugar fruit in it (for example celery juice, kale juice, wheat grass juice)

Low Sugar Alkaline & Keto Fruit:
- limes
- lemons
- grapefruits
- pomegranates
- blueberries

Fats & Oils
- Flax oil (not for cooking)
- Avocado oil (not for cooking)
- Hemp seed oil (not for cooking)
- Walnut oil (not for cooking)
- Expeller-pressed sesame oil (not for cooking)
- Duck fat
- Goose fat

Nuts & Seeds
- Flaxseed (raw, ground)
- Sesame seeds
- Tahini (sesame butter)
- Almonds (raw, soaked/sprouted)
- Almond butter
- Brazils (raw, soaked/sprouted)
- Hazelnuts (raw, soaked/sprouted)
- Pecans (raw, soaked/sprouted)

Alkaline Keto Food Lists & Recipes for Massive Weight Loss

- Pistachio Nuts (raw, soaked/sprouted)
- Walnuts (raw, soaked/sprouted)
- Macadamias (raw, soaked/sprouted)
- Macadamia butter
- Pine Nuts
- Pili nuts
- Chia seeds (raw and soaked)
- Nut flours - Coconut, almond

My Mediterranean grandma, who lived (enjoying excellent health) till 95 years old, used a lot of healthy food combinations from the lists above, for example:
-fresh salmon with a ton of green veggies, drizzled with organic olive oil (I can still remember how everyone would criticize her for "adding more fat," but she was adding good fat)
-hard-boiled eggs with fresh lettuce, tomato, avocado and olive oil, herbs and sea salt
-organic meat with a ton of leafy greens
-bone broths with good fats in it
-scrambled eggs, with herbs, butter, and leafy greens
-fresh tuna salad with olive oil and apple cider vinegar
-avocado salad with olive oil, herbs, sea salt, and lemon juice
-full-fat cheese with veggies, olives, and healthful oils...
I am getting hungry now when I look at that menu!

My grandma was also a fan of lemon-infused water, as well as adding a bit of apple cider vinegar to water and having it as a night drink. I do it all the time, it's a healthy habit to develop, and it helps reduce inflammation (inflammation is the root of all evil).
Ok, so now, after we have seen what is allowed on this lifestyle and how delicious it can get, let's focus on the second part of the food lists. Please note, it will not be hard to eliminate or reduce them,

after you have started adding the "freely allowed" foods. Give your body what it needs to thrive, and there will be less and less unwanted food cravings.

Foods to AVOID as much as possible:
Sugars, Sweeteners & Other
- White and brown sugar
- Coconut sugar
- Chocolate
- Raw honey
- Date syrup
- Pure maple syrup
- Molasses
- Tropical fruits
- Fruit juice
- Candy

Drinks
- Alcohol
- Caffeine
- A note about caffeine: 1, max 2 quality expresso a day is fine if you really need it. If you do, be sure to stay hydrated throughout the day. My delicious alkaline keto drinks from the recipe section will help you with that.

Other foods and drinks to avoid:
All commercial, refined, heat-treated, denatured, or artificial foods such as:
- bread
- baked goods
- sauces

- pastries,
- tinned foods
- microwave meals
- fast food
- breakfast cereals
- confectionery,
- sweets
- soy
- processed milk

Other:
All artificial sweeteners:
- Aspartame
- Sucralose
- acesulfame K
- saccharin
- xylitol
- sorbitol
- erythritol
- high-fructose corn syrup
- glucose
- fructose
- Golden syrup
- Agave syrup
- Rice malt syrup

Fats & Oils
All industrial seed oils such as:
- vegetable oil
- canola oil
- cottonseed oil

Alkaline Keto Food Lists & Recipes for Massive Weight Loss

- rapeseed oil
- corn oil
- sunflower oil
- hydrogenated oil
- safflower oil
- soybean oil
- peanut oil
- Non-extra virgin olive oils
- margarine and spreads
- Lard
- Shortening

Drinks
- All soda drinks, energy drinks, and diet sodas
- Commercial fruit juices and smoothies (even raw)
- Fruit cordials
- Milkshakes and flavored milk
- Artificial alcoholic beverages
- Soya milk

Fruits
- All fruit that is high in sugar

Grains
All grains, gluten, and flours:
- Wheat
- corn,
- rice
- spelt
- rye
- buckwheat
- barley
- oats
- bulgur

Other foods to avoid:
- beans
- lentils
- Peanuts
- Grain-fed meat and dairy
- All grains

- Soy
- Potatoes

If you haven't done so already, go to:
www.YourWellnessBooks.com/alkalineketo
to download and print your free alkaline keto food lists (as well as the lists of foods to avoid). As a bonus, you will also receive surprise gifts and other recommendations to help you on your journey!
Now that you have your alkaline keto food lists, we can move to recipe templates and meal plan ideas (followed by specific recipes). You have everything you need to start losing weight and feel amazing. I am thrilled (and so proud of you) that you have made it so far in this book!

Also, please note, now that you know what the alkaline diet and foods are. If you are feeling acidic, I would recommend you do a simple alkaline cleanse for a week or two and then jump on the alkaline keto bandwagon. An alkaline cleanse will help your body get rid of toxins, restore energy, and its natural ability to heal as well as to restore nutrients. While cleansing goes beyond the scope of this book, you can follow our #1 Alkaline Cleanse recommendation.

I go through this program once a year. It will help you eliminate sugar addiction, cleanse your body and get into an alkaline state to maximize your weight loss results (this program itself can help you lose weight within the next 2 weeks!).

You can learn more about it, in the recommended resources section at the end of this book.

Oh, and don't worry, the cleanse we recommend is not about going hungry. It's all about eating delicious, clean, and alkaline-rich meals to help your body get rid of fat and toxins and benefit from an alkaline keto lifestyle later on.

If you don't feel like you need a cleanse and your diet is already pretty clean and healthy, just dive right into the next sections!

Alkaline Keto Food Lists & Recipes for Massive Weight Loss

Alkaline Keto Meal Plans and Recipe Templates

Since we follow a simple, flexible, and stress-free approach, the recipes can be customized and arranged in an order that best suits you, your needs, and your lifestyle.

Some people thrive on 2 big meals a day and enjoy combining alkaline-keto lifestyle with intermittent fasting (for example, skipping breakfast or dinner).

A friend of mine is a big breakfast person, and he likes to wake up and have a massive alkaline keto breakfast, including eggs, bacon, avocados, and alkaline juice made of kale and grapefruits. Then, he has a late lunch consisting of cooked veggies or a massive salad with some fish or meat.

In the evening, he skips dinner and drinks lots of lemon water or green juice. This is his version of intermittent fasting, done in a flexible and customizable way.

Another friend of mine, who is a busy entrepreneur, starts her day with coffee (with some coconut oil or butter in it) and doesn't eat anything till lunch (she usually goes for a thick alkaline keto smoothie and some fish or tuna salad). In the afternoon, she has some green juice, and for dinner, she usually goes for some roasted veggies or a bowl of soup with some good fats and quality protein in it. It works great for her!

For me, well, I like to listen to my body and change things around, if needed. I can't eat too much at once, so having 2 massive meals a day doesn't cut it for me.

However, I also listen to my body. Sometimes, I just feel like skipping breakfast or dinner- my body is asking me to give its digestive system a rest. When you transition to a healthy lifestyle, you will be able to tune in and listen to your body- as it always tells you what you need. It works best when your diet is clean, and your focus is sharp (and there are no crappy carb or sugar temptations- when your body asks you for those, it means, it's out of balance, and it needs more good fats and alkaline foods to nourish and replenish itself).

So, please use the following sections in a flexible way. Some days include up to 5 meal suggestions. However, you can easily cut it down to 2 meals a day and intuitive fasting if you wish. Just be sure you eat enough calories during the day, even if you have only 2 meals a day.

We are focusing on clean foods and quality calories to give your body what it needs to lose weight – good fats and alkaline foods are our secret weapon. So why would we restrict it? It's supposed to help us.

Anyway, I will stop here, as the intro of this book, already covered the alkaline keto lifestyle to make sure you get the best results you could ever imagine, in a way that is fast but still healthy, balanced and fully sustainable!

Alkaline Keto Food Lists & Recipes for Massive Weight Loss

Day 1

-Wake up:
Drink lemon water with a little bit of Himalayan salt (you can also use some green powders; we have many great recommendations at:
www.YourWellnessBooks/resources)

If you drink coffee, you can enjoy quality espresso with 1 tablespoon coconut oil in it.

-Morning or Mid-Morning Smoothie:
Avocado, Coconut Milk, Chia Seeds, Coconut Oil, Stevia and Cinnamon

-Lunch:
Greens of your choice, tomato, tuna or smoked salmon, organic goat cheese, olive oil, and Himalayan salt

-Afternoon:
Smoothie (you can use your morning smoothie leftovers), or green juice (for example, arugula, parsley, grapefruit, avocado oil, and Himalayan salt).

-Evening:
Quality meat, or fish, with broccoli, cooked veggies or a salad (you can recycle your lunch salad)
Remember to drink lots of clean water (preferably alkaline water) during the day, in between your meals.
You can also drink herbal teas, such as fennel tea or red tea (great for weight loss or fat burn).

Day 2

-Wake up and make a green alkaline keto smoothie
For example:
Coconut milk, arugula leaves, coconut oil, a few slices of avocado and cucumber, a handful of cashews, plus some Himalayan salt and black pepper.

-Lunch: A simple "smoothie style soup":
Use the smoothie you made for breakfast and add in some meat or fish leftovers from your dinner. You can also add in some hard-boiled eggs.

-Afternoon:
A green powder drink, green tea with coconut oil, or quality expresso with coconut oil and coconut milk

-Evening: veggies cooked in coconut oil, with some cheese and Italian spices

Day 3

-Wake up and make breakfast:
Organic bacon and eggs, cooked in coconut oil or butter and served with a big bowl of leafy greens

-Lunch:
A simple, 3 ingredient salad, including tuna or smoked salmon, hard-boiled eggs, and fresh tomatoes, with olive or avocado oil, black pepper, and Himalayan salt.

-Afternoon:
Tomato juice (organic or homemade) with some avocado slices or nuts.

-Evening:
Spiralized zucchini cooked in coconut oil, spices, and homemade pesto (with some quality meat if you want).

The recipes are designed to be simple, quick, and easy to make, delicious, and filling!
Now, let's have a look at our recipe templates.

Alkaline Keto Salad Recipe Template

Option 1:
-1 cup of greens of your choice
-a few slices of smoked salmon, fried bacon, or some meat/fish leftovers (you can also use tuna, smoked chicken, smoked mackerel or sardines).
-tomatoes, cucumbers or any veggies of your choice
-olive or avocado oil, spices, and Himalayan salt

Option 2 Alkaline Keto Salads without Meat
-1 cup of greens of your choice
-half cup of chopped veggies of your choice
-half cup cheese slices
-hard-boiled eggs
-olive oil, avocado oil, Himalayan salt and spices

Option 3 Quick Tuna Salad Idea
-1 cup of greens or veggies of your choice
-1-2 cans of tuna
-olives
-cheese (optional) or avocado slices
-olive or avocado oil

Alkaline Keto Smoothie Template

-1 cup coconut or nut milk (unsweetened)
-1 tablespoon coconut oil
-avocado
-nuts or chia seeds
-half cup to 1 cup of greens
-low sugar fruits (grapefruits, limes, lemons, tomatoes).
-herbs and spices (cinnamon, stevia, and nutmeg for sweet smoothies; chili, salt, and pepper for spicy smoothies).

Alkaline Keto Juice and Drink Template (no juicer needed)

-1 or 2 limes, lemons or grapefruits – squeezed (you can use a lemon squeezer)
-1 cup coconut or nut milk
-1 tablespoon melted coconut oil
-1 cup herbal tea of your choice, cooled down, but still warm (lavender, mint, or fennel are my favorites)
Combine together, drink, and enjoy!

Warm Alkaline Keto Recipe Template

-greens or veggies of your choice
-a few slices of bacon, turkey or other quality, grass-fed meats- you can also use smoked salmon
-butter or coconut oil to cook/gently stir-fry
-onions and/or garlic
-Himalayan salt and spices of your choice

For example:
Heat up some coconut oil or butter in a frying pan (low or mid-heat).
Add your bacon/ or salmon/ or turkey slices
When almost ready, add in some spinach or veggies and cook until the veggies are soft.
Keep adding spices and salt to taste. Enjoy!

Alkaline Keto Chicken Broth Style Soup Template
Start boiling 2 -4 organic chicken legs.
Add in 5 garlic cloves (peeled), Himalayan salt, olive oil, and spices.
Keep cooking on high heat for about 40 minutes.
When the chicken gets tender, lower to low heat and add some veggies of your choice (for example, broccoli).
Keep cooking until ready, serve, and enjoy!

Now, that we are done with simple meal plans and recipe templates (to give you an idea of how you can easily combine different alkaline-keto ingredients to create delicious and balanced meals), let's have a look at some of my favorite alkaline keto recipes.

Alkaline Keto Recipes Made Super Easy!

Easy Low Carb Pizza Adventure

Yes, you heard me right. You can enjoy a healthy homemade pizza on this lifestyle. And...you can use it to add in some alkaline veggies too!

This recipe is just perfect for a lovely, lazy weekend evening when you're feeling cozy watching movies (keep the leftovers for the next day, pizza for breakfast, every now and then is also a great idea!). Please note- this recipe calls for a processed ingredient (tortillas). For me, personally, it's OK occasionally.

Servings: 2
Ingredients:
- 2 tablespoons coconut oil or organic butter
- 2 tablespoons olive oil
- 2 large low-carb, gluten-free tortillas
- 6 tablespoons organic tomato sauce (you can also make your own by blending 1 tomato with 1 tablespoon olive oil)
- 1 green bell pepper, minced
- 2 cans of natural tuna
- 1 cup shredded mozzarella cheese
- 4 teaspoons dried Italian seasoning
- Pinch of Himalaya salt

Instructions:
1. Using a large skillet (over medium-high heat) heat the coconut oil.
2. Add the tortilla.
3. Using a spoon, spread the tomato sauce over the tortilla.
4. Then, add the cheese, the seasonings, salt, tuna, and veggies.
5. Cook until crispy and then place on a cutting board and cut into thin slices.
6. Sprinkle with 1 tablespoon of organic olive oil on top.
7. Repeat the process to make more if needed.

Suggestions:
The possibilities are endless with this recipe. Feel free to experiment by adding veggies, greens, smoked salmon, some meat leftovers…whatever you want.

You can use all kinds of organic cheeses, veggies, and if desired, some meat or fish.

Irresistible Veggie Pizza

This is a delicious vegetable-based dish that combines the benefits of alkaline keto diets. It also calls for good fats while helping you enjoy the aroma and taste of cheese and Italian spices.

Servings: 4
Ingredients:
- 4 big zucchinis, peeled and cut lengthwise, very thin
- 4 tablespoons coconut oil
- 2 red bell peppers
- 2 green bell peppers
- 1 big onion, peeled and cut into thin rings
- 1 cup mushrooms, washed and sliced
- 1 cup mozzarella cheese powder
- Half cup organic tomato sauce (or blend 2 tomatoes with 2 tablespoons of olive oil to make your own)
- Himalayan salt
- 1 tablespoon oregano

Instructions:
1. Pre-heat the oven to 500 °Fahrenheit (or 260 °Celsius).
2. Grease a big, flat baking dish with coconut oil.
3. Add the zucchini and then the successive layers of red and green bell peppers, mushrooms and onions.
4. Sprinkle the cheese, salt, and oregano.
5. Place in the oven for about half an hour.
6. Serve and enjoy!

Easy Chili Tea

This tea will help in cleansing your digestive tract while warming you up and giving you a substantial energy boost that will last for hours.

Serves: 2

Ingredients:
- 2 cups water, boiling
- 2 Rooibos tea bags
- 2 red chili flakes
- A handful of fresh mint leaves
- 2 tablespoons coconut oil or organic butter

Instructions:
1. Place all the tea ingredients (except coconut oil) in a teapot and pour over 2 cups of boiling water.
2. Keep covered for 15 minutes.
3. Strain and serve warm (but not boiling) in a teacup with coconut oil or butter.

Cumin and Caraway Tea

This tea is excellent for women looking to obtain relief from period cramps. Adding in some good fats enhances the therapeutic properties of this alkaline keto style tea.

Serves: 1-2
Ingredients:
- 2 cups water, boiling
- 1-inch ginger, peeled
- 1 tablespoon cumin seeds
- 1 tablespoon caraway seeds
- 1 tablespoon coriander seeds
- 1 tablespoon fennel seeds
- 2 tablespoons coconut oil or avocado oil

Instructions:
1. Place all the tea ingredients (except the oil) in a teapot and pour over 2 cups of boiling water.
2. Keep covered for 15 minutes.
3. Strain and serve warm (but not boiling) in a teacup with the coconut or avocado oil.

Easy Flavored Spinach Juice

While pure spinach juice can be a bit hardcore, this recipe is a bit different.
Add in some fresh ginger and mix it with coconut milk and oil, and you will fall in love with green juice.
One green juice a day will keep the doctor away!

Serves: 2
Ingredients:
- 2 cups of fresh spinach
- 2-inch ginger, peeled
- 1 tablespoon melted coconut oil
- 1 cup of coconut milk

Instructions:
1. Place the spinach and ginger through a juicer.
2. Extract the juice, pour it in a big glass.
3. Combine with coconut milk and oil.
4. Stir well and enjoy.

Red Bell Pepper Antioxidant Juice

Red bell pepper, ginger, and healing greens is an excellent combination. It makes the juice taste nice and helps you get accustomed to juicing greens.

Servings: 2
Ingredients:
- 1 big red bell pepper, chopped
- 1 cup mixed greens of your choice (I like to throw in some spinach, arugula, and mint)
- 2 inch of ginger, peeled
- 2 tablespoons avocado or olive oil
- Himalaya salt to taste

Instructions:
1. Juice all the ingredients using a juicer.
2. Serve in a glass.
3. Enjoy!

Easy Chilly Beetroot Soup

This soup is creamy and comforting. It can be served warm, or raw and is a great way to recycle some meat or fish leftovers!

Servings: 2-3
Ingredients:

- 1 small avocado peeled and pitted
- 1 small beetroot, peeled and chopped
- 2 tablespoons of spring onion, chopped
- 1 small cucumber, peeled
- Half green apple, chopped
- 1 cup water, filtered, preferably alkaline
- Half cup almond or coconut milk

Toppings:

- Fresh dill, chive or herbs like oregano
- Meat or fish leftovers, or hard boiled-eggs, or avocado slices

Instructions:

1. Add all ingredients to blender.
2. Blend well until smooth.
3. Taste and adjust seasonings if needed. Blend together once again.
4. Serve (room temperature or chilled).
5. Add in some protein of your choice if you want.

Spicy Creamy Coconut Dream

This soup is just perfect if you enjoy spicy food. It's also great for detox!

Servings: 2
Ingredients:

- 2 tablespoons green onion, chopped
- 1 cup thick coconut milk
- 2 tablespoons of curry powder
- 1 minced garlic clove
- 2 small zucchinis, peeled and steamed
- 1 tablespoon grated ginger
- 1 handful cilantro
- 1 green bell pepper, chopped
- 1 small chili flake

Instructions:

1. Blend all the ingredients in a blender or a food processor.
2. Blend for 2 minutes to warm the soup.
3. Blend until creamy and smooth.
4. Garnish with cilantro.
5. Serve and enjoy!

This soup can be also served as a side dish to balance out animal products.

Anti-Inflammatory Ginger Soup

Ginger is alkaline, anti-inflammatory, anti-bacterial and it will make your soups taste spicy and delicious! Perfect alkaline-rich side dish to balance out the acid-forming effect of animal products.

Servings: 2
Ingredients:
- Half cup almonds, soaked in water for at least a few hours
- 1 cup coconut milk
- 2 tablespoons avocado or coconut oil
- Half cup water
- 2-inch ginger, peeled
- Half garlic clove
- 1 big cucumber, peeled
- Pinch of Himalaya salt and black pepper

Instructions:
1. Simply blend all the ingredients in a blender.
2. Serve in a soup bowl (room temperature, or chilled).
3. Enjoy!

Light Alkaline Keto Juice

This juice is particularly useful for healthy eyesight and beautiful skin as it is packed with Vitamins A and C.

It also helps fight inflammation and takes care of your liver.

Ingredients:
- 1 cup radish, cut into smaller pieces
- 5 celery stalks, chopped
- 1-inch ginger
- half lime, peeled
- 1 cup coconut milk
- 1 tablespoon sesame or flax seed oil
- Pinch of Himalayan salt

Instructions:
1. Juice the radish, ginger, lime, and fennel.
2. Pour into a glass.
3. Add in the Himalayan salt and oil.
4. Stir in the coconut milk.
5. Stir well, serve and enjoy!

Apple Cider Antioxidant Juice for Optimal Energy

This recipe is full of miraculous nutrients to help you get rid of toxins. Its therapeutic properties are enhanced by Apple Cider Vinegar.

Servings: 1-2
Ingredients:
- 2 cucumbers, peeled and sliced
- Half cup of celery leaves
- Half cup of mint leaves
- 2 tablespoons of olive oil
- 1 tablespoon apple cider vinegar (organic)
- Himalayan salt to taste (optional)

Instructions:
1. Juice all the ingredients.
2. Add in the olive oil, apple cider vinegar, Himalayan salt, and black pepper.
3. Serve and enjoy!

If your goal is weight loss and body detoxification, you can start adding about 1-2 tablespoons (a day) of quality, organic, apple cider vinegar to your alkaline-keto drinks.

Apple cider vinegar goes really well with therapeutic alkaline keto juices (and also smoothies). It's inexpensive and very effective.

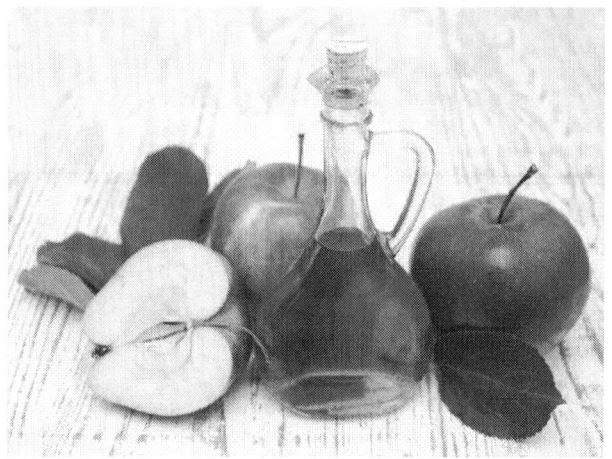

Herbal Weight Loss Juice

This recipe fuses the low sugar alkaline fruits with horsetail infusion. Horsetail infusion is an excellent natural remedy to get rid of water retention, lose weight, and burn fat. It's full of alkaline minerals and blends really well with this juice.

Ingredients:
- A handful of fresh mint leaves
- A handful of celery leaves
- 1 grapefruit, cut into smaller pieces
- A green apple, cut into smaller pieces
- 1 lime, peeled
- Half inch ginger, peeled
- 1 cucumber, peeled and cut into smaller pieces
- Half cup horsetail infusion cooled down
- Optional: stevia to sweeten

Instructions:
1. First, juice all the ingredients.
2. Pour into a glass.
3. Combine with horsetail infusion. Add stevia if needed.
4. Serve and enjoy!

Amazing Keto Chocolate Shake

Who said that a healthy lifestyle means no desserts? You can enjoy desserts in a homemade, healthy, clean version. You have already learned how to make super healthy salads and smoothies, and it's all great. But we only live once, and so whenever you crave a shake, enjoy this one! No sugars, no nasty chemicals...

Servings: 2

Ingredients
- 1 cup heavy (whipping) cream, or coconut cream (no added sugar)
- Half cup coconut milk (or almond milk) unsweetened
- 1 teaspoon stevia
- Half teaspoon maca powder
- Half teaspoon vanilla extract
- 4 tablespoons unsweetened cocoa powder

Instructions:
1. Pour the cream into a chilled metal bowl.
2. Start beating the cream with a hand mixer.
3. Keep beating until it forms peaks.
4. Stir in the coconut milk.
5. Proceed to add stevia, maca, cocoa, and vanilla powder.
6. Beat again until the mixture is thoroughly combined.
7. Pour into shake classes and chill in a fridge for a couple of hours.
8. Serve and enjoy!

Suggestions: you can serve the shake with some protein powder or chia seeds.

Ridiculously Easy Sweet Alkaline Keto Balls

This recipe is a must-try to help you:
-satisfy your "sweet tooth" without eating crappy carbs or sugars
-add in some good fats and anti-inflammatory properties too
-sneak in some alkaline keto superfoods to make sure you stay energized

Ingredients:
- 1 cup raw cashews (unsalted, unsweetened), soaked for at least 4 hours
- 1 cup raw almonds (unsalted, unsweetened), soaked for at least 4 hours
- 4 tablespoons coconut oil
- 4 tablespoons coconut milk
- 1 tablespoon cinnamon powder

Instructions:
1. Place all the ingredients in a high-speed blender or a food processor.
2. Using your hands, form the "dough" into small balls.
3. Place the balls on a big plate and put in a fridge for a few hours.
4. Serve and enjoy!

Creamy Sweet Alkaline Keto Porridge

This recipe is perfect if you are craving something sweet and creamy. It's super easy to make.

Servings: 2
Ingredients:
- 1 cup raw cashews
- 1 cup of coconut milk
- 2 tablespoons coconut oil
- 1 tablespoon cinnamon powder
- 1 tablespoon chia seeds
- Optional: 1 teaspoon maca powder
- A few blueberries to garnish

Instructions:
1. Combine all the ingredients in a bowl.
2. Mix well, serve and enjoy!

Smoked Salmon Green Salad

This salad offers another filling lunch option. Horseradish cream spices it up and gives it a unique flavor.

This salad is perfect as a takeaway lunch that will keep you full until the late afternoon or early evening.

Serves: 2
Ingredients:
- 4 big slices of smoked salmon, cut into smaller pieces
- 1 teaspoon of horseradish cream
- 3 large organic tomatoes, sliced
- 2 small cucumbers, peeled and sliced
- ½ cup of coconut yogurt
- 1 cup fresh watercress
- Juice of 1 lemon
- A dash of ground black pepper
- Himalayan salt to taste

Instructions:
1. Place all the ingredients into a salad bowl. Stir well.
2. Season with black pepper and Himalayan salt to taste.
3. Enjoy!

Easy Mediterranean Baby Spinach Salad

Spinach is rich in essential alkaline minerals and protein as well as high iron content.

Serves: 1-2

Ingredients:
- 1 cup of raw baby spinach
- 1 cup of raw zucchini, grated
- Half cup of raw cherry tomatoes halved
- A handful of black olives, pitted and halved
- A handful of green olives, pitted and halved

Dressing Ingredients:
- 2 tablespoons of extra virgin olive oil
- Juice of 1 lime
- 2 small garlic cloves
- 1 chili flake
- Pinch of Himalaya salt
- Pinch of black pepper
- 3 segments of orange
- 3 tablespoons thick coconut milk

Instructions:
1. Start off by blending all the dressing ingredients using a blender.
2. Place the raw baby spinach onto a serving plate.
3. Top with the grated zucchini and cherry tomatoes.
4. Add the black and green olives.
5. Pour over the salsa and toss well.
6. Drizzle with the olive oil and serve.

Cucumber Creamy Green Smoothie

This is one of my favorite "on the go" smoothie recipes as it doesn't require that many ingredients. Thanks to the cucumbers, It's full of alkaline minerals and very hydrating.

Servings: 2

Ingredients:
- 2 big cucumbers, peeled and roughly sliced
- 1 cup full-fat coconut milk (unsweetened)
- Pinch of Himalaya salt to taste
- Pinch of black pepper to taste
- 6 radishes, sliced
- 2 tablespoons chive, chopped

Instructions:
1. Place the cucumbers, and coconut milk in a blender.
2. Add the Himalaya salt and black pepper.
3. Blend well and pour into a smoothie glass or a small soup bowl.
4. Add in the radishes and chive.
5. Mix well and add more Himalaya salt and black pepper if needed.
6. Sprinkle the cheese and enjoy!

Boost Your Brain Smoothie

The flaxseed meal is an excellent source of Omega-3 fatty acids, aka "good fats". After having this smoothie, not only will you feel full and satisfied but you will also get an energy boost!

Serves: 1-2

Ingredients
- 1 big avocado, washed and pitted
- 1 cup of almond milk,
- 2 teaspoons of flaxseed meal
- A handful of fresh baby spinach, washed
- Optional: 1 teaspoon fresh moringa powder
- Optional: half cup filtered water or coconut water, if needed

Instructions
1. Place all ingredients in a blender.
2. Blend until combined and almonds are blitzed.
3. Serve in a chilled glass and enjoy!

Cheesy Pumpkin Surprise

The combo of pumpkin and cilantro, along with the pine nuts, and other spices, makes this salad incredibly flavorful.
Organic mozzarella cheese makes this salad taste amazing!

Serves: 2-3
Ingredients:
- Half cup of fresh cilantro, well rinsed and dried with a kitchen towel
- A handful of fresh parsley, well rinsed and dried with a kitchen towel
- 1 cup of pumpkin, cooked, peeled and finely sliced
- Half cup of fresh cherry tomatoes, halved
- A few slices of fresh mozzarella cheese, cut into smaller pieces
- Half cup of raw pine nuts

For the Dressing:
- 1 teaspoon of nutmeg powder
- 1 teaspoon of curry powder
- ¼ teaspoon of Himalaya salt to taste
- 1 tablespoon of sesame seed oil

Instructions:
1. Place the fresh cilantro and parsley in a serving bowl.
2. Top with the pumpkin, mozzarella, and cherry tomatoes.
3. Add the raw pine nuts and sprinkle the spices and salt over the top
4. Drizzle with the sesame seed oil and serve.
5. Enjoy!

Alkaline Green Keto Energy Salad

Turn to this quick, detox salad whenever you need to increase your energy levels! It's fast, natural, tasty, and effective.

Serves: 2-3

Ingredients:
- 1 cup fresh baby spinach leaves
- 1 raw green sweet pepper, sliced
- 1 cup raw cherry tomatoes, halved
- 1 big orange, peeled and segmented
- ¼ cup raw pistachios, roughly chopped
- 1 big ripe avocado, peeled, pitted and sliced
- 2 tablespoons avocado oil

Instructions:
1. Place the baby spinach in a serving bowl.
2. Top with the rest of the ingredients.
3. Add the raw pistachios.
4. Drizzle with the avocado oil, serve.

Healing Herbs Avocado Salad

The herbs used in this salad make avocado taste amazing, and they also add to the mineral and nutrient content of this salad.

Serves: 2
Ingredients
For the Salad:
- 2 avocados, peeled, halved and pitted
- ¼ cup of mixed Mediterranean herbs (for example thyme, rosemary, basil, oregano, parsley)
- ¼ cup of dried cherry tomatoes, quartered
- ¼ cup of cooked turkey or chicken
- Optional: 1 sheet of nori, cut into smaller pieces

For the Dressing:
- 1 tablespoon of extra virgin avocado oil
- Juice of a half lemon
- Pinch of black pepper and Himalaya salt to taste, if needed

Instructions:
1. Place the avocado halves in a serving bowl.
2. Add the rest of the ingredients.
3. Drizzle with some avocado oil and lemon juice.
4. If needed, season with Himalaya salt and black pepper.
5. Enjoy!

Ketoricious Energy Smoothie

This recipe uses hemp oil, which is great to re-balance hormones, soothe anxiety and improve the mood.

Serves 1-2

Ingredients
- 1 tablespoon of hemp oil
- 1 cup coconut milk
- 1 avocado, pitted and peeled
- A handful of cilantro leaves, washed
- 1 teaspoon spirulina
- Pinch of Himalayan salt
- Pinch of curry powder
- Optional (if you like it spicy) a pinch of chili powder

Instructions
1. Place all the ingredients in a blender.
2. Process until smooth.
3. Taste to check if you like to taste or if you need to add a bit more of Himalayan salt or curry powder
4. Serve in a smoothie glass, or a bowl and enjoy!

Herbal Wellness Smoothie

This smoothie is great for digestion and relaxation. It also helps prevent sugar cravings.

Serves 1-2
Ingredients
- 1 tablespoon of mint leaves
- 2 tablespoons of coconut oil
- ½ cup of cashew milk
- ½ teaspoon of fresh vanilla
- ½ cup chamomile infusion, cooled

Instructions
1. Place cashew milk, mint leaves and vanilla in a blender.
2. Process until smooth.
3. Pour into a smoothie glass and mix it with chamomile infusion (warm or cold, depending on your preferences).
4. Enjoy!

Please note – cashew milk can be replaced with almond milk, coconut milk, or any nut or plant-based milk of your choice. Just make sure there is no added sugar.

The Supermodel Glow Smoothie

Good fats from avocado and coconut oil will help you stay full longer and prevent sugar cravings. It will help you have a glowing, healthy looking skin too! All this while helping your body get back to balance.

Serves 1-2
Ingredients
- 1 tablespoon coconut oil
- 1 cup of cashew or other nut milk of your choice
- 2 small zucchini, steamed and peeled
- 1 big tomato
- Handful of fresh cilantro leaves, washed
- 1 teaspoon moringa powder

Instructions
1. Place all the ingredients in a blender.
2. Process until smooth.
3. Pour into a smoothie glass, stir well, serve and enjoy!

Easy Spicy Papaya Salad

The combination of spicy chili really compliments the sweetness of the papaya in this recipe. The cashew nuts add a really nice crunch and a hearty dose of protein.

Serves: 1
Ingredients
For the Salad:
- 3 tablespoons of Mediterranean herbs mix
- 1 cup of diced fresh papaya
- 4 fresh cucumbers, finely sliced
- Half teaspoon of fresh red chili powder
- A handful of raw cashew nuts, roughly chopped

For the Dressing:
- 1 tablespoon of virgin olive oil
- A pinch of Himalayan salt

Instructions:
1. Place herbs in a serving bowl.
2. Top with the cucumber, papaya, and cashews.
3. Sprinkle the chopped chili and coconut shavings over the top and toss together.
4. Drizzle with the olive oil and serve.
5. Enjoy!

More Alkaline Keto Books

Questions?
You can email me at:
info@yourwellnessbooks.com

Alkaline Ketogenic Lifestyle for Massive Weight Loss is the sixth book in the *Alkaline Keto Diet Book* series.

The first book in the series is called: *Alkaline Ketogenic Mix*: *Quick, Easy, and Delicious Recipes & Tips for Natural Weight Loss and a Healthy Lifestyle.*

It's a step-by-step beginner guide to help you transition to a healthy alkaline-keto way of eating without feeling deprived.

Other books in the *Alkaline Keto* series focus on specific recipes or cooking methods, for example: *Alkaline Ketogenic Salads*, *Alkaline Ketogenic Smoothies & Juices*, or *Alkaline Ketogenic Green Smoothies.*

There is no recommended reading order – feel free to pick up your next alkaline keto book by focusing on your favorite recipes, or a specific alkaline keto cooking method you wish to dive deeper into (for example salads or smoothies).

You will find all the Alkaline Keto Diet books on Amazon & listed on our website. You will also find them by searching for "Alkaline Keto Elena Garcia" on the Amazon website (US or other countries).

www.amazon.com/author/elenagarcia
www.yourwellnessbooks.com/books

More Alkaline Keto Books

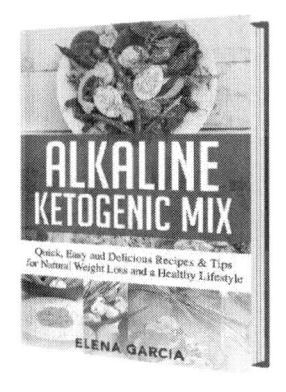

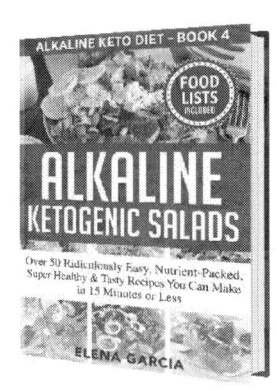

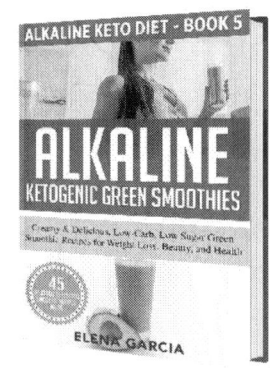

(FYI, there is also a romance/erotica writer who uses the name Elena Garcia on Amazon, however, it's not me. I only write wellness and weight loss as well as healthy eating books!).

By searching for Alkaline Keto Elena Garcia, you will be able to find other books in the series.

If you are looking for specific alkaline keto supplements, programs, or other tools and brand recommendations (readers ask me all the time), I have listed everything on our website to help you save your research time:

www.YourWellnessBooks.com

Extra Resources to Help You on Your Weight Loss Journey

1. Alkaline Acid Charts available at:

www.YourWellnessBooks.com/charts

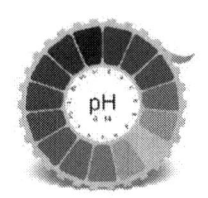

2. Recommended - Alkaline Plant-Based Cleanse – discover how to lose weight and get rid of sugar cravings without feeling hungry or deprived:

www.YourWellnessBooks.com/cleanse

3. Alkaline water recommendations:

www.YourWellnessBooks.com/alkalinewater

4. Alkaline Keto Food lists:

www.YourWellnessBooks.com/alkalineketo

We Need Your Help

One more thing, before you go, could you please do us a quick favor?

It would be great if you could leave us a short review on Amazon.

Don't worry, it doesn't have to be long. One sentence is enough.

Let others know your favorite recipes and who you think this book can help.

Your review can inspire more and more people to turn to the alkaline ketogenic lifestyle so that they can finally achieve their wellness and weight loss goals the way they deserve.

Your honest review is critical.

Thank You for your support!

Join Our VIP Readers' Newsletter to Boost Your Wellbeing

Would you like to be notified about our new health and wellness books? How about receiving them at deeply discounted prices?

What about awesome giveaways, latest health tips, and motivation?

If that is something you are interested in, please visit the link below to join our newsletter:

www.yourwellnessbooks.com/email-newsletter

As a bonus, you will receive a free complimentary eBook *Alkaline Paleo Superfoods*

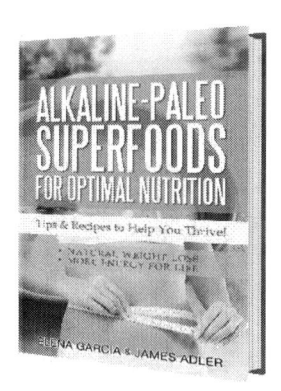

Sign up link:

www.yourwellnessbooks.com/email-newsletter

More Alkaline Keto Books

More Books & Resources in the Healthy Lifestyle Series
Available at:

www.yourwellnessbooks.com

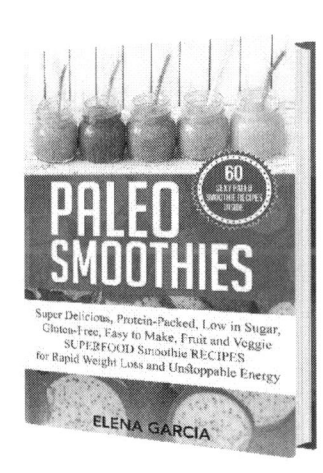

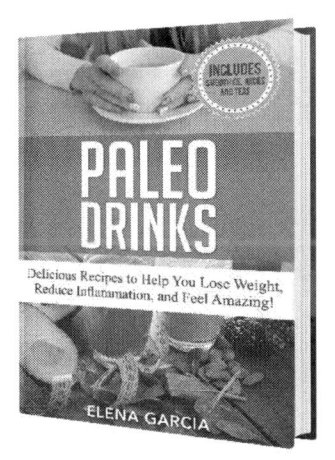

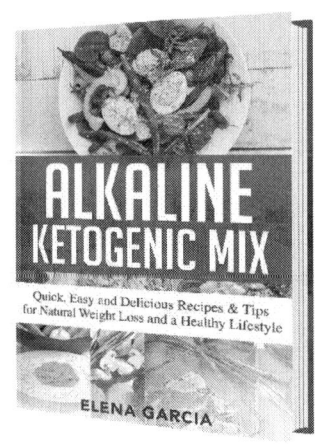

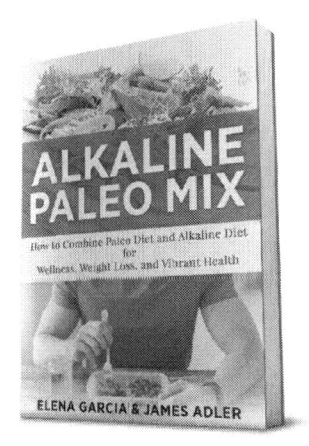

More Alkaline Keto Books

Until next time, wishing you all the best on your journey!

Elena & Your Wellness Books Team

Manufactured by Amazon.ca
Bolton, ON